Save Your Life
With the Elixir of Water

Becoming pH Balanced in an Unbalanced World

by

Blythe Ayne, Ph.D.

Save Your Life
With the Elixir of Water

Becoming pH Balanced in an Unbalanced World

by

Blythe Ayne, Ph.D.

Save Your Life with the Elixir of Water
Becoming pH Balanced in an Unbalanced World

Blythe Ayne, Ph.D.

Emerson & Tilman, Publishers
129 Pendleton Way #55
Washougal, WA 98671

*Book & cover design by Blythe Ayne
Thank you to Pixabay for the gorgeous Public Domain photos
Image of Nebraska Sunset – © Blythe Ayne*

Save Your Life with the Elixir of Water
Becoming pH Balanced in an Unbalanced World

Other books in the save your life series:
Save Your Life With The Power of pH Balance
Save Your life with the Phenomenal Lemon (And Lime!)
Save Your Life With Stupendous Spices

www.BlytheAyne.com

Paperback ISBN: 978-1-947151-55-0

*1. HEALTH & FITNESS/Diet & Nutrition/Nutrition
2. HEALTH & FITNESS/Healing
3. HEALTH & FITNESS/Diseases/General*

BIC: FM
Second Edition

E&T

DEDICATION:

To All Who Seek Knowledge, Truth, & Excellent Health

Table of Contents

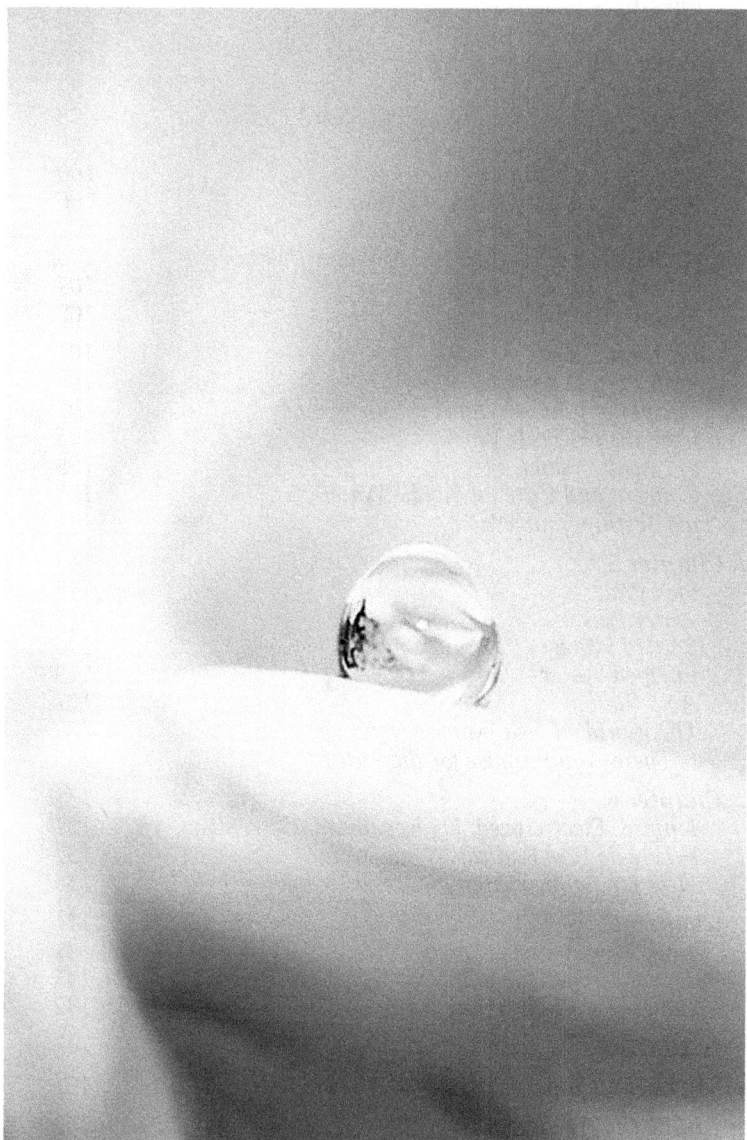

Chapter 1:
You & Water

"Water is the driving force of all nature."
Leonardo da Vinci

What are You?

Aside from being an Amazing Being, what are you? Well, physically, you're 60 to 70 percent water. Your tissues and organs are predominately made of water. Your brain is 75 to 90 percent water, your heart is 75 percent water, your blood is 90 percent water, your eyes are 90 percent water, your lungs are 85 percent water, your skin is 72 percent water, your muscles and kidneys are 75 to 80 percent water. Your beautiful, solid bones are 30 percent water. Your liver, an amazing 96 percent water, uses that water to metabolize fat, (which, interestingly, is only 10 percent water), into energy.

A human embryo is over 80 percent water. A newborn baby is 74 percent water.

Medical science is taking notice of the tremendous ability of the human body to heal with adequate, healthy water. Your body does know how best to heal, and how to support healthy longevity. Water is central to every aspect of good health.

The Rivers of Life in You
Water is the mode of transportation in your body. Fuel from the foods you eat is transported by your water-dominant blood to your hungry cells, while the waste of every cell's metabolism is carried away. The plasma, which, again, is 90 percent water, passes through your arteries and veins, accomplishing all the myriad tasks of an extremely active and continuous transit system—working energetically Every. Single. Moment.

Stay Hydrated
Recall the tin woodsman in The Wizard of Oz, rusted into stasis, muttering through rusted-shut jaws, "oil can."

Your heart, your liver, your spleen, your kidneys, your stomach, your intestines, all the rest of your organs, your bones, your muscles, your skin, your hair, your eyelashes, your toenails, your fingernails, your eyes, your teeth, your nerves, your brain, your brain synapses—in short, every bit of you, every minute of every day, cries out for hydration if you're not drinking enough water.

Water is human oil. (And oil for all other creatures and plants, as well.)

Water lubricates every joint and runs every chemical function for each little cell to get all the nutrients it needs, as the lovely river of water passes through your body, while taking with it all the toxins and waste, to flush them out.

The wide Mississippi, the mighty Columbia, the peaceful Nile, the powerful Amazon, the spiritual Ganges, the ancient Tigris and Euphrates are the arteries of civilization, depositing rich nutrients along the way and carrying off toxic wastes. But if they're over-taxed, their effectiveness rapidly diminishes.

The rivers in you are exactly the same. Flowing through your arteries, bringing good health to all the thirsty "lands" along your arteries, and taking downstream the pollutants, contaminants, and toxins.

The Water You Drink Becomes YOU!

"A river seems a magic thing.
A magic, moving, living part
Of the very earth itself."
Laura Gilpin

The Science of Water

Water is involved in every metabolic process, every electrical exchange, every biochemical pathway, in short, every physical and mental action, every breath you take, every move you make, that makes you "YOU!" Water extracts nutrients from food and transports these nutrients to the blood, water replenishes vital fluids, and water is central to the processes that detoxify your body.

Without adequate water your body must recycle what it already has, re-filtering this depleted water through your kidneys, placing an extra burden on your kidneys and your liver.

Water's Journey

After leaving the stomach, water is absorbed mostly in the small intestine, while some water absorption occurs in the stomach and the colon. The absorption process is very rapid—studies show that water appears in plasma and blood cells as soon as 5 minutes after ingestion![1]

Water passes from the intestinal lumen (the cells in the spaces between tissues), into plasma, and is then distributed via blood circulation all over the body.

Water moves freely into the interstitial fluid, across cell membranes via water specific channels. The body's water is renewed dependent upon the quantity of water ingested: the more reliably you hydrate, the more your body's water is renewed.

Here's an example of water's journey for a man drinking eight cups of water per day: a molecule of water will stay in his body about ten days, with 99 percent of the body's water renewed within 50 days.

Dehydration

Herman Aihara, father of modern Macrobiotics, noted that we have an inner sea of saline fluid that carries nutrients, energy, messages, and, yes, toxins to every part of the body. Then this inner sea carries away the toxic elements and wastes in its numerous, ever-working, metabolic processes.

The osmotic flow of water through the cells' membranes generates hydroelectric energy, used by all the body's cellular processes, including neurotransmission. All runs smoothly as long as there's enough water.

But trouble begins when there is not enough water. When your body does not receive enough hydration to perform its myriad, amazing processes, it puts into operation a priority rationing and distribution system for the inadequate amount of water that's available.

Dehydration has a very serious negative effect on your body's cells. When your body is dehydrated, the distance across the membrane of your cells changes, becoming longer, and, as a result, the substances that need to go through a cell's membrane begin to get stuck in it. Toxins and metabolic waste accumulate in these changed body cells and cannot leave the body.

Your body simply can't function normally if its cells are damaged. When the transportation of oxygen and nutrients through the body slows down, pain and disease is the result. To be twenty percent dehydrated is life threatening.

A Few Harmful Effects of Dehydration:
• Tiredness
• Migraine
• Constipation
• Muscle cramps
• Irregular blood pressure
• Kidney problems
• Dry skin
• The list goes on

Symptoms of Dehydration
Dry Skin: Your skin is your largest organ and requires a lot of water. If you have dry skin, you need more water.

Thirst: If you feel thirsty, you're already dehydrated. It's always a good practice to drink water when you're not thirsty. Don't wait!

Hunger: Many people mistake what they think are hunger cues as a sign to eat more, when in fact, they may be dehydrated. So before you sit down to your meal, drink a glass of water (though it is advised not to drink water during the meal, as it interferes with the process of digesting food, "watering down" the digestive enzymes).

Fatigue: If you're fatigued, drink one or two glasses of water. It's refreshing and will give you a boost in energy.

Fluid Retention

The first thing the body does when it becomes dehydrated is retain fluids. Your body must store water if you do not provide enough, or if it is unusually tapped when demands are made on body water during periods of illness—diarrhea, vomiting, fever, an intense work out, or intense period of physical labor, in addition to medical problems such as congestive heart failure, kidney malfunction, protein deficiency, hormonal imbalance—all make demands on body fluids.

One of the most common causes of fluid retention is sodium (salt) retention. As sodium retains water in a specific, unalterable concentration, fluids will be retained to maintain this dilution. But as additional water, free of sodium, is introduced, your body will be able to eliminate the excess sodium. Therefore, drink more water to get rid of excess water!

Water pills abnormally force water out of the body, thus the problem of water retention has not been solved for the long term. Also, since the primary function of the colon is to reabsorb water, an inadequate amount of water means a nearly complete reabsorption of available fluid, with the result of severe constipation.

Fluid retention is your desert-body's desperate effort to survive. To reiterate, if you want to eliminate fluid retention, drink more water, not less.

Dehydration causes chronic pain. Abdominal pain, ulcers, constipation, colitis, joint pain, back pain, low energy, mental confusion, disorientation, and a myriad other health issues are the result of the concentration of acids and toxins recirculating in the depleted water. Pain is the consequence of the drying interfacial tissue (the layer right under the skin), causing friction and inflammation. The interfacial tissues must be lubricated to be lubricating.

The lymphatic fluids, central to our immune system, remove wastes from the body. But when we don't have enough lymphatic fluids, the body becomes extremely toxic. This toxicity leads to disease. The organs, and all the systems throughout the body, become impaired if they don't receive adequate nutrients from blood, and if they aren't cleansed by the lymphatic fluids.

If you're not drinking enough water for your body to make healthy, clean blood to distribute nutrients and to perform the necessary removal of toxins, you have made a perfect environment for disease.

> *Fluid retention is your body's*
> *desperate effort to survive.*
> *To eliminate fluid retention*
> *drink more water!*

It Doesn't Get Better

When there is nutritional, electrical, structural, toxicological, or biological imbalance in the body, microforms flourish. Healing chronic illness can only take place when and if the blood is consistently maintained at a normal, slightly alkaline, pH.

We live in a world-wide plague of yeasts, fungi, viruses, and molds inhabiting our bodies, depositing their excretions. Toxic wastes are produced when they consume the glucose, fats, and proteins the body needs, stealing our food, turning it into poison, then, adding insult to injury, dumping their poisonous wastes inside of us.

Mitochondria are the body's cellular power plant, and our entire metabolic process depends upon the mitochondria being in balance. Your seventy-five trillion (75,000,000,000,000) cells are slightly acidic within, with their health entirely dependent upon the interstitial fluid surrounding them being slightly alkaline.

Without this delicate acid-alkaline pH balance, chemical and energy interchanges cannot occur. The pH opposites—acid and alkaline—are the means by which electricity flows in your body. There must be a perfect polarity between the interior of a cell and the fluid surrounding it, or the cell's energy cannot flow into the surrounding tissues.

We can survive days without food, but four days without water can be fatal. Water is more than a carrier of other materials. And as we contemplate how much we love water, let us take into consideration all these other actions, processes, and procedures water performs for us, for all creatures, for plants, and for Mother Earth, herself.

Water is:
- a nutrient transport system
- an electrical message system
- an energy combustion system
- a waste disposal system
- a chemical conduit
- a lubricant
- a solvent
- a dilutor
- a dilator
- a coolant
- a latent heat bank

And, if you've studied with Masaru Emoto, (featured in **What the Bleep Do We Know?**) as I had the great fortune to do, you know that he taught that water is the repository of emotion.

Well, hmmm, if overall we're seventy percent water, and our brains are 90 percent water, where else, exactly would our emotions be, but in water?

> *"Everywhere water is a thing of beauty*
> *gleaming in the dewdrop,*
> *singing in the summer rain."*
> **John Ballantine Gough**

Seductive Liquid Poisons

Drinking anything other than water is not the same as drinking water.

Alcohol, coffee, soft drinks, even fruit juices, have substances that are not healthy, undoing the positive effects of the water they contain.

Coffee, caffeinated beverages, sodas, and tea (depending on the type), act as diuretics, depleting the body of urgently-needed water, and stimulating the adrenal glands, which leads to adrenal fatigue. A cola is ten-thousand times more acidic than your blood. We mistake our over-stimulated adrenal glands as a signal of quenched thirst and a boost of energy. It could not be further from the truth.

Soft drinks also contain sodium, and phosphorus which depletes bone calcium. A twelve-ounce can of soda has the equivalent of nine teaspoons of sugar—all those empty calories, without any fiber, that water has to figure out what to do with.

Fruit juices, even natural, "no sugar added" fruit juices, contain the fruit's sugar, stimulating the pancreas.

Drinking beverages other than water, to the virtual exclusion of water, causes people—especially children—to lose their taste for water, becoming dependent on sodas and juices. This is a critically unhealthy "addiction."

Drink More Water to Prevent Inflammation

Most people are not drinking enough water. Instead, they're drinking coffee, alcohol, fruit juices, sodas and bottled water. Bottled water is generally very acidic. All of these substances, without the benefit of pure, alkaline water, damage the body over time.

Dehydration from these "not water" beverages has a compounding effect. With dehydration comes inflammation. Inflammation manifests in many medical conditions: high blood pressure, obesity, pain, anxiety, depression, asthma, high cholesterol, arthritis, so on and so forth.

Besides the life-threatening diseases that are fostered by chronic dehydration, mild to moderate dehydration manifests problems as well: headaches, migraines, diminished memory, muddy thinking, low energy, depressed mood, irritability, frustration, sadness.

These conditions are augmented by the very process of treating them with drugs.

For example, if you take an over-the-counter medication for a headache caused by dehydration, you put an even greater strain on your body, as that headache medication is acidic. Your dehydrated body is already battling an overly-acidic condition driven by inadequate water, increasing the oxidative stress throughout your body, and increasing inflammation.

This is a vicious cycle that makes you even more thirsty.

This vicious cycle applies to most pharmaceuticals as well, as they are acidic, stressing the body's systems. All of this magnifies the effects of dehydration.

Long term dehydration and inflammation weakens your immune system, making you more susceptible to the damage caused by viruses, which means staying sick longer.

Drink Water Before You're Thirsty

By the time you think, "hmmm, I'm thirsty," you're already dehydrated. And, further, the sensation of a dry mouth is a sign of extreme dehydration. As your body works to adjust to long term deprivation of water, the thirst mechanism becomes disabled.

The result is a decreasing thirst sensation over time, with the obvious consequence of increased dehydration. As you give your body more water, the thirst mechanism begins to work again, but it may not become apparent until your body is fully hydrated.

You'll discover that when you're actually drinking enough water, you're often thirsty! In fact, that's how you'll know you are supplying your amazing body the water it needs—when you frequently become aware of its request for water.

How Much is Enough?

It's commonly cited that the minimal amount of water is eight 8-ounce glasses—that's 64 ounces—of water per day, If you're not there yet, increase your intake gradually, until you've established a habit of this minimal amount of water. Two 32-ounce bottles per day is another way of looking at it.

An athletic, or otherwise highly active person needs to increase daily water consumption to 12 to 14 cups of water. The more you exercise the more water you expend and the more you need to replace.

There's a phenomenon known as "breakthrough," when you've finally established a daily habit of 8-12 glasses of water, all the stored water is released, and the stagnant, retained fluid is flushed.

In addition to numerous other benefits, you'll discover that you're thirsty and have a desire to drink the amount of water your body needs as a regular habit. The thought, "I have to drink at least 64 ounces of water," will shift to, "I'm thirsty! Time for my water."

Maintaining this level of water intake solves the problem of fluid retention, and will reflect glowingly in your general improved health, and, last but not least, will significantly contribute to weight loss. For every 25 pounds you exceed your ideal weight, increase your daily intake of water by an additional eight ounces.

Dr. Batmanghelidj, author of Your Body's Many Cries for Water, gives this advice: "Balance your sodium intake with your water consumption. Add 1/4 teaspoon of Celtic sea salt or Himalayan sea salt per quart of water."

Many people believe that their anxiety, depression, inflammation, high blood pressure, joint pain, head-aches, and other disease processes need to be treated with medication. But so many of these conditions would be reversed—let alone never manifest in the fist place!—if people simply drank enough healthy water.

Stay Hydrated!

> *"When the well is dry,*
> *They know the worth of water."*
> **Benjamin Franklin**

Science & Chemistry
Water is the medium for the multitude of enzyme and chemical activities in any body regardless of species. Water moves nutrients, hormones, antibodies, and oxygen through the bloodstream and lymphatic system, into cells. Proteins and enzymes of the body function more efficiently in solutions of lower viscos-

ity—less "stickiness." Water is the body's solvent, regulating all bodily functions, including everything it dissolves and everything it circulates.

Every cell in your body needs water. For example, as your brain is 90 percent water, if it is inadequately watered, you will experience fatigue, confusion, forgetfulness, headaches, migraine, and/or brain fog. As little as a two percent drop in the amount of water in your body can bring on mental confusion, short-term memory loss, and an inability to focus.

When you experience any of these symptoms of dehydration, immediately drink one or two glasses of water.

Your Body's Use of Water
An adult human body uses approximately three quarts (six pints/twelve cups) of water every day. About 56 percent, (over three pints), of water is used and filtered out of your body through your kidneys, 20 percent (one to two pints) through your lungs from simply breathing, 20 percent (one to two pints) dissipates through your skin, and four percent is used by your gastrointestinal tract. Four ounces of water dissipates daily through the soles of your feet.

You also need water to breathe—the delicate membranes of your respiratory tree must have adequate moisture for the exchange of gases in the lungs. As we take in oxygen and excrete CO_2, our lungs must be moistened by water. One to two pints of water is used every day in the basic, life sustaining process of breathing.

Water is the lubricant for your joints.

More than one gallon of water per day is used for your intestinal absorption, with 90 percent being reabsorbed by the colon.

Water regulates body temperature. A hot day or strenuous physical activity can cause a significant increase in demand on your body's water, as much as a quart per-hour to cool your body by evaporation through the skin. This water loss must be replaced.

Energy
Your energy is affected by the amount of water you drink. A mere five percent drop in body fluids will cause you to lose up to 30 percent of your energy. A 20 percent drop in body fluids can cause the body to shut down altogether. Yes, this is dire. We must constantly replace the water that is used by bodily functions, activities, and environmental conditions.

Organs and systems throughout your body will be damaged if they aren't cleansed by lymphatic fluids—which are part of the immune system and remove wastes from the body. When you don't drink enough water for your body to produce these lymphatic fluids and healthy blood, you set yourself up for disease.

Your blood pumps through your heart at approximately 275 pints (130 liters) per hour. Your kidneys filter two pints (one liter) of blood per minute. When the kidneys become clogged with wastes, kidney stones develop, and the bladder becomes inflamed.

All of the blood in your body is filtered of toxic wastes and acids as it passes in the bloodstream through your liver every three minutes. And that's not the liver's only job—it also produces enzymes that alkalize the blood, keeping it in perfect pH balance.

When liver function tests show an elevation of enzymes, the liver is being taxed to work overtime to reduce excessive toxins and acid wastes. When attending to the acid imbalance, the liver cannot appropriately address its other functions, and must sort out what to do with excess wastes. So it deposits the wastes in joints, just to get the acids away from the more vulnerable and critical life-supporting organs. The result is arthritis, along with all the other "-itises," and fibromyalgia, and the like.

Respiration—breathing—is another means of alkalizing the blood. Oxygen sustains the alkaline environment in the body, which is why yoga, tai chi, and other movement-focusing-on-the-breath exercises are so beneficial for your health. They support healthy, limber joints, and the added oxygen contributes to alkalizing and detoxifying your body. Drinking water while exercising is yet more beneficial.

Your body uses the alkaline minerals, calcium and magnesium, working in conjunction with one another, to buffer acidity. When the body is overly acidic, it will "steal" calcium from teeth and bones—resulting in tooth decay and osteoporosis. Osteoporosis is not a lack of dairy products, but rather an overabundance of acids, which can be neutralized by adequate water.

When the body is properly alkalized, these concerns do not arise.

Stress is another factor in the body's excessive use of magnesium and calcium, as stress is acid-producing. Depleted magnesium and calcium cause us to stress more readily. Yes, you're very observant—this is yet another vicious-cycle- downward-spiral.

But you can make it a happy-cycle-upward-spiral by becoming more hydrated. Try drinking one or two glasses of water when stressed.

Drink your anti-stress water mindfully. Become calm. Release the stress. Simply Stop.

Be. In. The. Moment.

Other uses—and forms—of water that are beneficial in reducing acidity are steams and saunas, allowing your largest organ, the skin, to flush out toxins. Oh, happy body!

What Produces Acids?

Let's first keep in mind the broad categories of alkalizing components:
• Water
• Fruits
• Vegetables
• Mindful eating
• Calming exercise
• Meditation
• Deep breathing

Now the acidic components:
• Alcohol
• Drugs—licit and illicit
• Smoking
• Junk foods
• Inadequate chewing
• Being sedentary
• Toxic environment
• Physical stress
• Emotional stress
• Over-processed foods (long lists of ingredients on packaged food)
• Shallow breathing (make a habit of breathing deeply, into your stomach)
• All animal products—meat, dairy, and eggs

Simple formula:
- Drink water
- Eat a plant-based diet
- Take vitamin B12 and vitamin D supplements.

> *"I came where the river*
> *Ran over stones;*
> *And all the waters*
> *Of all the streams*
> *Sang in my veins*
> *That summer day."*
> **Theodore Roethke, The Waking**

She Blinded Me with Science!

How does your body create energy? It creates energy when your cells remove electrons from amino acids, sugars, and fatty acids from your food to add those electrons to other molecules, especially oxygen. With this process, unstable particles—free radicals—are created. They are highly reactive, and if there are too many of them, they will cause cellular damage, also known as oxidative stress.

If you've been reading carefully (or you may already know), you've seen that free radicals manifest during the normal functioning of your body. They are produced from digestion, when you exercise, when you're out in the sun, when you're exposed to the physical stress of pollution, and when you're mentally/emotionally stressed from your job, relationships, family and life events.

So it's normal and unavoidable to have free radicals. Under reasonable conditions, your body will create enzymes to clean them up before they cause cellular damage. But we're dealing with more free radicals than our bodies can cope with due to excessive stress, excessive pollution, excessive acidic diets, and inadequate exercise, with the resultant cellular damage, and the resultant life-taking diseases, in the prime of so many people's lives.

It's heart-breaking. Millions of people are essentially committing suicide without realizing it.

My goal is that you fully realize the outcome of your choices, and, when necessary, make different choices!

More Blinding Science
Any beverage or food that provides an extra ion is an antioxidant. An ion is energy, and when the extra ion is given to an unstable oxygen molecule, also known as a free radical, that unstable oxygen molecule is neutralized—stabilized—by the ion. Once neutralized, the now-stabilized molecule can be absorbed by a cell and used for energy.

But if the free radical stays unstable, that is to say, is not provided with an antioxidant, alkaline ion, it continues to bounce around in the cell, damaging it.

Years of excessive free radical damage deteriorates cells, which leads to disease.

The Details

Your body requires a minimum of 90 different nutrients to maintain ideal health. Nutrients that act as antioxidants include: vitamin C, beta carotene, selenium, phytochemicals and flavonoids (the biologically active compounds in plants). Some antioxidants are enzymes that our body creates, one such enzyme is superoxide dismutase.

If your body fluids are acid, that is to say, positively charged, they are flowing about, looking for alkaline (negatively charged OH- ion) materials to react with. The nutritionally important alkaline minerals include: calcium (Ca+), magnesium (Mg+), potassium (K+), sodium (Na+), zinc, and iron, found in your liver, muscles, ligaments, teeth, bones, etcetera.

Meanwhile, the alkaline, negatively charged minerals are drawn to the H+ ion, acid minerals, which include: chlorine (Cl-), sulfur (S-), phosphorus (P-). They form hydrochloric acid (HCl), sulfuric acid (H2SO4), and phosphoric acid (H3PO4).

The goal is always to produce a pH balance. The seriousness of pH imbalance is driven by:
1. excessive acids on the planet
2. excessive acids in animal-based foods
3. excessive acids in over-processed foods
4. excessive acidic bodily response to life stresses

Once again: acidic pH is the result of an acid-forming diet, emotional stress, toxic overload, immune reactions, or any process that deprives your cells of oxygen and other nutrients. The body works to temper acidic pH by using alkaline minerals. A diet with inadequate alkaline minerals leads to a build-up of acids in cell walls referred to as acidosis.

Acidosis causes, aids, and abets:
cardiovascular damage/weight gain/obesity/diabetes / bladder problems/constipation / diarrhea/kidney stones/immune deficiency/acceleration of free radical damage / hormonal problems/premature aging/osteoporosis/joint pain/aching muscles/ lactic acid buildup/low energy/chronic fatigue/ slow digestion/slow elimination/yeast/fungal overgrowth/lack of energy/lower body temperature/ tendency to get infections/loss of drive, joy, enthusiasm / depression/easily stressed / pale complexion / headaches/migraines/inflammation of the corneas, eyelids/loose, painful teeth/ inflamed, sensitive gums/mouth ulcers /stomach ulcers / cracks at the corners of the lips / excess stomach acid / gastritis / thin nails / hair falls out, has split ends / dry skin / skin easily irritated/leg cramps, spasms—and more.

Your Body's Metabolism
All the body's fluids are slightly alkaline: the interstitial fluid, the cerebrospinal fluid, the

lymphatic fluid, liver bile, and so forth. The only exception is the hydrochloric acid produced, when needed, in the stomach to process the materials that come into it, so they can be used for adequate fuel.

Your body is slightly alkaline, but cells produce acid as a by-product when doing their work. In a clockwork functioning, healthy body, the acid waste produced is reduced to carbon dioxide and water, which we naturally breathe and flush out.

It's a beautiful and amazing flow! Think about it—at this very moment, your body is in the midst of a-million-and-one activities, from its own impeccable knowing, without you having to direct a single bit of it.

But to go a little deeper (though not too deep) ... not every bit of what you eat is completely metabolized. There's a residue that's referred to as ash. The digestive process oxidizes food with enzymes that break down your food into alkaline ash and acidic ash.

An interesting example of alkaline ash is lemon. Although acidic in its raw state, it burns to an alkaline ash, which consists of mineral salts: sodium, potassium, calcium, etcetera, making it one of nature's healthiest foods (for more—a lot more—on this "miracle fruit," read my book, *Save Your Life with the Phenomenal Lemon & Lime*[2].

Most other fruits and vegetables are alkaline and burn alkaline.

Meanwhile, protein-based foods, (and this is categorically all animal products), burn to an acid ash consisting of phosphates, sulphates, and nitrates (from the phosphorus, sulphur and nitrogen in proteins). In a world that is already over-acidic, acid-ash foods need to be limited.

Acid ash cannot be eliminated through the lungs as carbon dioxide and water in the same way as in the previously discussed cellular metabolism. Your body must buffer the acid ash with its precious store of alkaline substances, that is to say, sequester the acid ash, to neutralize it. In no case is this good. This buffering takes place both inside and outside of cells, with the majority of the buffering occurring in the blood itself.

The paramount importance of drinking alkaline water becomes ever-more obvious.

In order to reduce the acidity of the blood, the lungs remove carbon dioxide (CO_2), and expel it through breathing. Carbonic acid (H_2CO_3) becomes water (H_2O) when carbon dioxide is removed, which is the fastest way to reduce blood acidity. The pH value of blood in the veins fluctuates widely depending upon the waste products dumped into them. That's why the artery blood pH value is used as a reference—in order to survive, it must remain at pH 7.365.

"How beautiful is the rain!
After the dust and the heat,
In the broad and fiery street,
In the narrow lane,
How beautiful is the rain!"
Henry Wadsworth Longfellow, Rain in Summer

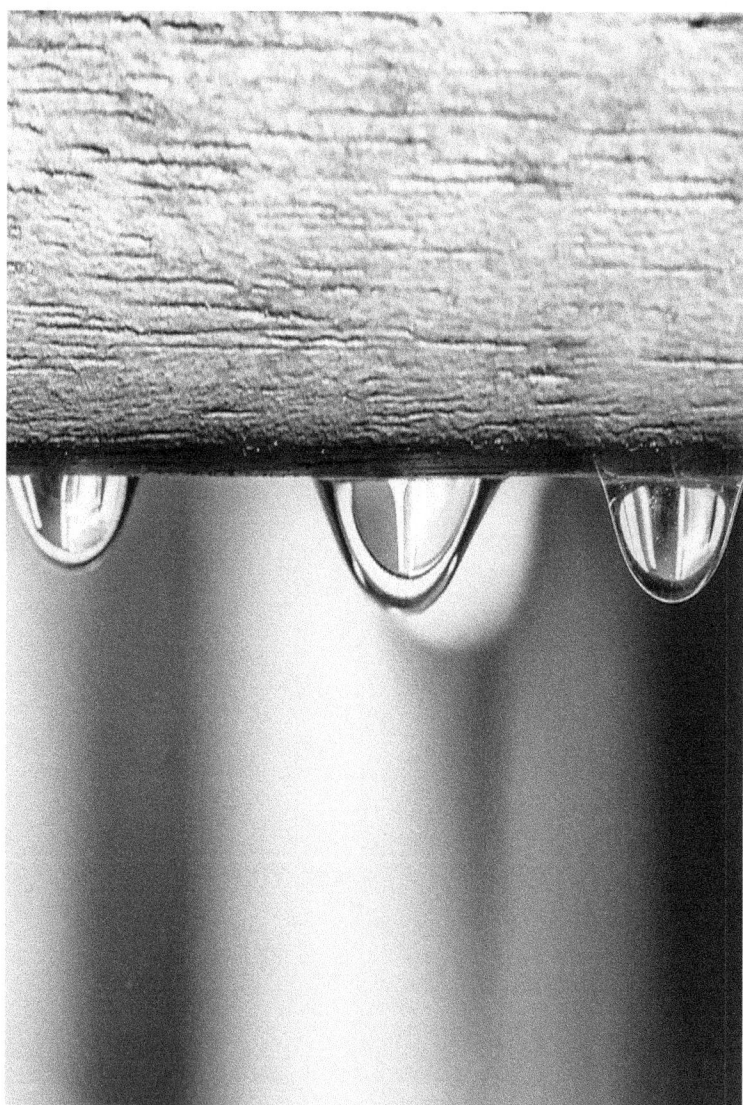

Chapter 2:
The Water in You —
From Head to Toe

The Circulatory System

*H*umans have a closed blood circulatory system, meaning it does not leave the network of arteries, veins, and capillaries. The components of the human cardiovascular, or circulatory, system are the heart, blood and blood vessels including pulmonary circulation, which is a loop through the lungs oxygenating the blood, and the systemic circulation, a loop through the rest of the body to provide it with oxygenated blood.

The circulatory system circulates blood, which transports oxygen, carbon dioxide, hormones and nutrients—such as amino acids, electrolytes, and blood cells—to and from the cells in the body. This process provides nourishment, assists in finding diseases, stabilizes body temperature, stabilizes pH, and just generally maintains homeostasis.

Although our cardiovascular system is closed, oxygen and nutrients diffuse across the blood vessel layers, entering the interstitial fluid, carrying oxygen and nutrients to cells, while removing carbon dioxide and wastes, as mentioned.

Components of Blood

The average adult has five to six quarts of blood, roughly seven percent of one's body weight. Blood consists of plasma, red blood cells, white blood cells, and platelets. Plasma, which is 55 percent of your blood, is 90 percent water. The remaining ten percent is glucose, mineral ions, hormones, used-up proteins, and carbon dioxide.

Red blood cells, which are made in your bone marrow, account for the other 45 percent of the blood. In red blood cells, hemoglobin, a protein, carries oxygen throughout the body. The other job of red blood cells is to remove carbon dioxide, carrying it to the lungs to exhale.

White blood cells, also produced in the bone marrow, are your immune system, protecting against disease and foreign invaders. And last but not least, blood contains platelets, whose job it is to stop bleeding by clumping and clotting the blood.

Patently obvious is the importance of adequate hydration to keep the blood rich and healthy for its many life-sustaining responsibilities.

The circulatory system also includes the lymphatic system, discussed in the next section.

"Next to blood relationships,
Come water relationships."
Stanley Crawford

The Lymph System

The lymph system is generally under-appreciated, even though so profoundly important. It's dependent upon you to keep it healthy, and to exercise every day. A simple walk will make your lymphatic system very content. It has no heart to provide circulation—the "motor" for the lymph system to cycle is you, in motion. When you exercise, your muscles expand and contract—this drives the lymphatic fluids, which must have plenty of healthy water and a healthy, alkaline diet.

What the Lymph System Is

There are between six hundred and seven hundred lymph glands in your body! It's a network of lymphatic vessels, lymph capillaries, lymph nodes and organs, lymphatic tissues and circulating lymph. Lymph is recycled blood plasma—it has been filtered from the interstitial fluid, and returned to the lymphatic system.

What the Lymph System Does

The lymph system:
• fights infections
• recycles plasma proteins

• filters the lymph
• drains fluid back into the venous circulatory system from the tissues to prevent dehydration

Like plasma, lymph is 90 percent water. It's made up of two components:

1. white blood cells and lymphocytes that attack bacteria in the blood, and

2. chyle—fluid from the intestines containing proteins and fats.

Your body has approximately 2.4 to 3 gallons of lymph, which is twice the volume of blood (1.2 to 1.5 gallons), and twice as many lymph vessels as blood vessels. Lymph fluid carries nutrition to the cells and removes acid wastes, combating viruses, bacteria, cancer cells, heart disease, arthritis, and other threats to your health and life.

When the body is overly acidic, the lymph system, which needs an alkaline environment to flow freely, slows down. Gradually, acids are stored in tissues and the lymph dries, forming adhesions throughout the tissues.

These adhesions interfere with the flow of both lymph fluid and blood. Waste products from foods incompletely or improperly digested due to an acidic imbalance, are reabsorbed into circulation via the lymphatic ducts of the small intestine. Poisons that are not daily cleared via the bowels are reabsorbed into the body.

The solution to prevent tissue adhesions and the reabsorption of waste poisons back into the body? As always, a healthy, alkaline diet and plenty of water.

Keep your lymph system's rivers and streams well watered!

The Digestive System

The human digestive system, which is dependent upon the presence of adequate water, includes the gastrointestinal tract, salivary glands, pancreas, liver, gallbladder, tongue, teeth and epiglottis. The process of digestion has many stages, which begins in the mouth. It involves the breakdown of food into smaller and smaller components, until they can be absorbed and assimilated into the body.

Chewing food mixes it with saliva, which contains a catalytic enzyme called amylase. This begins the process of digestion. Another digestive enzyme, lingual lipase, is secreted by lingual papillae on the tongue and serous glands in the salivary glands. Food then travels down the esophagus into the stomach. Here it mixes with gastric juices, then passes into the duodenum to mix with enzymes produced by the pancreas.

The largest structure of the digestive system is the gastrointestinal tract (GI tract), which is about thirty feet long. Yes, thirty feet. Keep that in mind when you ingest acidic foods and beverages that do not digest fully, putrefying in that thirty feet of gastrointestinal tract for days. (Fruits, vegetables, and alkaline water trip merrily through the thirty feet in hours, in a healthy manner.)

Most of the digestion of food takes place in the small intestine, while the largest part of the GI tract, the large intestine, absorbs much-needed water, to keep the waste matter in motion, headed for the exit.

The colon must be kept clean of accumulated acid wastes. Poisons and excess acidic wastes collect on the colon walls. These cause diarrhea and constipation, and harden, then are re-absorbed into the bloodstream. Not good! Regular, healthy bowel action is an indicator of a healthy, alkaline, diet.

Aging & Anti-Aging

Aging is driven by the accumulation of acidic wastes in the body.

Here's the acid-driving list again: acidic diet, over-eating, inadequate water, mentally and/or physically over-working, or, conversely, sedentary lifestyle (find the balance!), inadequate sleep, environmental pollution, drugs and alcohol, emotional stress, and smoking (don't smoke!). When all of these acidic irritants reach a critical mass, the body cannot get rid of all the accumulated acidic wastes. This makes you age. To maintain alkalinity in its fluids to survive, the body will convert some of the irritating liquid acid into solid acids such as fatty acids, uric acid, kidney stones, gallstones, urates, phosphates, and cholesterol (which comes only from animal products—meats, dairy, and eggs).

The excess of acidic wastes causes the blood to coagulate, it clogs capillaries, and prevents smooth blood circulation. The organs begin to have numerous problems when healthy blood circulation is compromised, and aging symptoms appear.

How it Works
The body burns nutrients in the cells to function. The main ingredients of all foods, whether gourmet or junk food, alkaline or acid, are:
- carbohydrates
- proteins
- fats

which are composed of four elements:
- carbon
- nitrogen
- hydrogen
- oxygen

After these nutrients are burned, i.e., oxidized, they turn into organic acids such as carbonic acids, uric acids, lactic acids, fatty acids, and ammonia. (It might be interesting to note that fats are acidic even before oxidation.) Mixed with these organic acids are inorganic acid minerals: chlorine, phosphorus, and sulfur that accompany acidic foods. Without a diet of anti-aging, alkaline foods that contain inorganic alkaline minerals: calcium, magnesium, sodium, and potassium, an alkaline pH balance cannot occur.

Aging & Acidosis

There's an obvious and direct relationship between aging and the accumulation of acids, i.e., acidosis. Therefore, please mindfully attend to the addition of alkalinity and the reduction of acidity to your body. Considering the whole body, there needs to be a net gain of alkalinity. In short, alkaline water is an easy and effective component of anti-aging.

When living with a compromised, acidic waste disposal system for a long period of time, some parts of the body build up more acids than others, clogging the capillary vessels in those acidic areas. This causes some organs to function sluggishly, which results in feeling tired and run down.

Feeling run down for seemingly no apparent reason can be mystifying, but it's because of a pH imbalance. Then diseases such as high blood pressure, arthritis, diabetes, asthma, allergies, and others, start to set in. Do not quietly accept these symptoms and diseases as simply "getting old."

Further, if pH balance is not well maintained, taking supplements such as vitamins, minerals, and trace minerals is a waste of money and supplements, because the body cannot absorb them in an acidic environment, and, instead, throws the supplements out, unabsorbed.

I return to my chorus: the solution to combat the diseases of aging is to be adequately hydrated. Unhappily, this fail-safe solution is entirely too simple for many people—including many allopathic doctors—to accept.

However, in response to the gathering body of scientific documentation that aging and disease are the direct result of the accumulation of acid waste products in the body, a growing number of health care practitioners and scientists are supporting a pH balanced lifestyle.

Help is On the Way

The help you need will come from none other than your *self*. This infallible help only requires two steps to put into effect:

1. Develop a healthy disposal system. The body's perspiration and elimination systems must have adequate water.

2. Pull out all the old, decaying, wastes from their nooks and crannies. This happens naturally with a healthy disposal system.

When step two has been accomplished, then all you need to do is attentively continue with step one.

It's practically miraculous how the organs will recover once healthy blood circulation is restored. You can halt, and even, it has been shown, reverse the aging process.

One For-Instance of Anti-Aging— How to Have Healthy Hair

Gray, dull, thinning hair is caused by oxidation, and oxidation is caused by free radicals. If you want to stop your hair from being oxidized, you need to neutralize the free radicals attacking your hair follicles.

There are people in their sixties, seventies, eighties, and beyond, who have amazing hair. Here are the things that healthy-hair people have in common: they are active—exercise helps eliminate toxins out of the body. They have diets that are high in vegetables and fruits and low in proteins, oils, salts, preservatives. They eat fewer calories than most people, which also lessens the strain on their body. They drink lots of healthy, alkaline, water.

The combination of exercise, fewer calories, fruit and vegetable diet, and plenty of water allows the body to perform at its optimum, and provides all the antioxidants needed to scavenge free radicals. The result? Beautiful hair, beautiful skin, beautiful smile! Beautiful, long life!

Enzymes

Superoxide dismutase, amylase, and catalase, are amazing and important enzymes. They clean up free radicals at a one-million to one ratio among our cells. Free radicals are unstable oxygen molecules bounding around inside cells and gradually breaking them down. It's important for free radicals to be cleaned up by these hard-working enzymes.

As we age, our body becomes less able to produce enzymes. Fewer enzymes obviously results in more free radical damage to our cells. But plenty of alkaline water makes an enzyme-friendly environment.

You Can Become Younger if You So Desire

The Brain
Brain tissue is 85 percent water. Although the brain is only one-fiftieth of your body weight, it uses one-twentieth of your body's blood supply. If your blood is water-deprived, the ability of the brain to generate energy and to function properly is sorely compromised.

The brain has a dual blood supply that comes from arteries. The anterior circulation arises from the internal carotid arteries, and supplies the front of the brain, the posterior circulation arises from the vertebral arteries, and supplies the back of the brain and the brainstem. The circulation from the front and the back join together at the circle of Willis within the brain.

Brain Dehydration
Even mild dehydration is associated with anger, depression, and confusion according to researchers

from Tufts University, Medford, MA. A study at King's College in London found that long periods of dehydration impairs brain functions, for example: spatial relations and the ability to plan.

Dehydration leads to stress, and stress manifests further dehydration.

Dehydration plays a major role in causing migraines. Migraine headaches may also be an indicator of critical body temperature regulation due to "heat stress."

Boosts Mood, Creativity & Work Productivity
As your brain is mostly made up of water, drinking more of it helps you think better, concentrate better, be more alert, and maintain an emotional even keel.

Always keep water within reach in your workspace—and everywhere!—stay hydrated to stay alert, and to resist the temptation to drink less healthy beverages. Remember that caffeinated beverages are diuretics and add to dehydration.

Eyes
Eighty percent of all information comes into the human brain through the eyes. Between the cornea and the iris, and between the iris and the lens are two cavities filled with the aqueous humor—which is 98 percent water.

Aqueous humor helps maintain eye shape, aids eyesight by providing support for the internal structures, and supplies nutrients, amino acids, and glucose to the lens and the cornea, while it removes the eye's cellular waste.

The eyeball itself is filled with vitreous humor which is 99 percent water. It has no cells, but is made up of small fibers. The functions of the vitreous is to transmit light to the retina, and to exert pressure against the retinal layers to keep them in place and functioning properly. It keeps the round shape of the eyeball, which is necessary for the lens to focus sharp images on the retina.

Each eye is encased in a pyramid-shaped bone structure. This is serious protection for the two delicate globes of essentially water, that provide you with the world you perceive.

To keep these optical miracles—your eyes—well-watered with healthy, alkaline water must be of the highest priority in your life.

Drink Plenty of Water
To Support Your Eyes & Your Sight

Teeth
Teeth are made of, predominately, enamel, and are the hardest substance in the body. They are only about four percent water.

However, water is extremely important for the health of your teeth, as it flushes away acids and sugars from their surfaces. Acidic foods on the teeth break down the enamel and sugary foods attract bacteria. Drinking water after a meal helps to prevent both of these actions that contribute to tooth decay.

Also, frequent water intake helps prevent the staining of teeth by coffee, tea, other beverages and foods such as berries.

Drinking lots of water helps keep your breath fresh by eliminating the environment in which bacteria—the cause of dry mouth and bad breath—thrive.

Hearing

The inner ear contains perilymph, made of sodium salts and water and endolymph fluids, made of predominately potassium and water. Pure, clean, alkaline water in drinking and in bathing is essential for hearing health.

Think about this: for eons humans had to live near a source of water—a lake, pond, stream, river, or ocean—in order to survive. People bathed in ponds. Drank water from streams. And to be clean, they submerged themselves in natural, clean, antioxidant, alkaline, bodies of water.

In our modern, rush-rush, hurry up, only-have-time-for-a-quick-shower world, some people are rarely, if ever, entirely submerged in clean water (acidic, chlorinated public pools do not count!).

Submerging in a clean alkaline bath allows for the release of toxins in a relaxed, rejuvenating state, while—bonus!—water passively hydrates the ears. This prevents the impacted build-up of dirt and toxins that leads to compromised hearing and eventually damages the inner ear's delicate bones.

For added benefit, pour a cup of Epsom salts in the bath, providing a topical application of much-needed magnesium.

If you have a jetted tub, that's even better on two counts: one, the moving, aerated water produces beneficial negative ions, and two, the gentle massage of the pulsations of water against your stressed, tired, dehydrated, muscles allows for yet more release of toxins and lactic acid build-up.

> *"The best thing one can do*
> *when it is raining,*
> *Is to let it rain."*
> **Henry Wadsworth Longfellow**

Heart

Your heart is one of the most alkaline-dependent organs in your body, partly supplied by the vagus nerve, which also functions best in an alkaline environment. Acid wastes actually alter the heartbeat, robbing the blood of adequate oxygenation, which, woefully but not surprisingly, degenerates the heart.

To state the obvious, an alkaline system creates ideal heart function.

Stay Hydrated!

In the United States, 610,000 deaths occur annually from heart disease. It's estimated that a habit of drinking an optimal amount of water could reduce the cardiovascular disease mortality rate by as much as fifteen percent, as suggested by the Safe Drinking Water Committee of the National Academy of Sciences.

Beware of "Soft" Water

There is a correlation between soft water, water with a pH below 6.5, and cardiovascular disease. The process of softening water (or purifying or distilling water), removes from the water much needed trace minerals, such as magnesium and calcium, that keeps it alkaline. Softened water is acidic, and augments the incidence of cardiovascular disease (among a plethora of other negatives).

Again, cells, tissues, and organs do not thrive in an acidic environment. They'll do anything to buffer this acidity, including removing minerals from your bones, and producing bicarbonate in the blood.

Do not drink distilled/purified/soft water. You will develop mineral deficiencies, which takes a serious toll on your health.

> "Our bodies are composed of the same minerals that form the sun and moon. Our hearts are rhythmically tuned to the pulsations of gold and white light that these wonders of God splash so abundantly across the porch of the mind."
> **Dr. Theodore Baroody**

Stomach, Pancreas & Intestines
Acid indigestion? Before grabbing an antacid, drink down a glass or two of water. Keep in mind that water is more alkaline than the acid you're battling and it will neutralize the acid.

Notice how most, if not all, of your acidic discomfort simply fades away. Acid indigestion is stressful, so while you drink your alkaline water, consciously become calm, center in your body, and relax.

Your Microbiome
We depend on a thriving microbiota for our health and survival. The home of microbes is in the small intestine, where much of the body's water and nutrients are absorbed. It must have adequate alkaline water to support the microbiome. Thus, an alkaline diet feeds the protective microbiota, to maintain a healthy acidic gut.

Certain bacteria, the anaerobes (microorganisms that require an oxygen-free environment), thrive best in a negatively charged, high alkaline environment. This alkaline environment supports the growth of lactic acid bacteria such as lactobacilli and bifidobacteria, which guard against the overgrowth of toxin-producing aerobes (microorganisms that require oxygen).

Aerobes in the small intestine lead to malabsorption syndrome, which prevents the absorption of nutrients, associated with serious diseases such as diabetes, obesity, cancer and neurodegenerative disease. Pathogenic bacteria such as E. coli thrive in an aerobic environment.

Peyer's Patches

The Peyer's Patches, essential for proper assimilation of food and for producing lymphocytes for the lymph system's nodal network, are in the upper portion of the small intestines. In addition to producing lymphocytes, they also produce large amounts of the alkalizing enzyme, chyle.

It's critical to have a steady flow of chyle into the lymph system to keep it alkaline. When there is too much acid waste from acid-forming foods, the Peyer's Patches cannot produce adequate chyle, thus compromising the entire system.

Break it Down!

The stomach produces acid when it needs to break foods down. In order to digest food and kill the bacteria and viruses that come with it, the inside of the stomach is very acidic, with a pH value that hovers around 4.

When we eat alkaline food and drink alkaline water, the pH value inside the stomach goes up. This commands the stomach wall to secrete hydrochloric acid to bring the pH value back to 4, so the stomach maintains its acidic environment.

The byproduct of hydrochloric acid is alkaline sodium bicarbonate ($NaHCO_3$) or potassium bicarbonate ($KHCO_3$), which goes into the blood stream. These alkaline bicarbonates neutralize excess acids in the blood, dissolving solid acid wastes into liquid form, alkalizing and detoxifying the body. As the alkaline bicarbonates neutralize the solid acidic wastes, carbon dioxide is released, which is discharged through the lungs.

Without the alkaline minerals in alkaline bicarbonate, the body becomes overly acidic, leading to acidosis. Acidosis in its mild form causes body aches, headaches, poor sleep, poor digestion, depression. If allow it to become more severe, acidosis is the precursor of serious diseases.

A Bit More Detail ....

When the stomach pH value gets higher than 4 (less acidic), the stomach generates hydrochloric acid to lower it back to 4. But if the pH value becomes more acid than 4 (a pH value less than 4), the stomach cannot produce hydrochloric acid, and produces acidic stomach gas pain instead, which is your intelligent body's clear signal that your stomach is being made too acidic.

What do people do? Reach for an antacid, which is merely palliative, not a cure. It's much healthier to drink a glass or two of alkaline water. When the stomach does not produce hydrochloric acid—which, again, it doesn't when it's too acidic—there is subsequently no production, or inadequate production, of alkaline sodium bicarbonate to go into your blood stream to neutralize the excess acids in the blood.

After the food in your stomach is digested, it moves into the small intestine so acidic it will damage the intestine wall. Pancreas to the rescue! All aspects of pancreatic function work toward reducing excess acidity and regulating blood sugar balance. To maintain proper blood sugar, you must provide the pancreas with a primarily alkaline-forming diet.

The pancreas makes alkaline pancreatic juice, (sodium bicarbonate), that mixes with the acidic food coming out of the stomach. In order to produce bicarbonates, the pancreas must make hydrochloric acid, which goes into the blood stream.

A careful reader will observe in the previous two sentences that the pancreas makes an alkaline product, and an acidic product. Its exocrine enzymes (alkaline) connect to the small intestine, its endocrine hormones (acidic) connect directly through the blood and nervous systems.

Do you not see what an amazing mechanism, what a perfect balance, what a dance with chemistry and nature, your miraculous, astounding, body is? All of this non-stop intelligence, going on within you—how can you not want to contribute to its perfection with alkaline water, alkaline diet, and less stress?

The most accessible of these, of course, is *WATER*.

Other Organs

Here are thumbnail sketches of a few of the other organs, and their dependence upon water:

Lungs

Your lungs are about 83 percent water. Gas exchange occurs in the lungs, whereby CO_2 is released from the blood, and oxygen is absorbed.

In a bit more detail, in order to reduce the acidity of the blood, the lungs remove carbon dioxide (CO_2), and expel it through breathing. Carbonic acid (H_2CO_3) becomes water (H_2O) when carbon dioxide is removed, which is the body's fastest way to reduce blood acidity.

Oxygen-depleted blood is pumped away from the heart via the pulmonary artery to the lungs, then the pulmonary vein returns the oxygen-rich blood to the left atrium.

Bronchial circulation, a separate system, supplies blood to the tissue of the larger airways of the lungs.

The Liver

Your liver is an amazing 96 percent water, and has over three hundred functions. It processes acid toxins from the blood and produces numerous alkaline enzymes. Your liver is your first line of defense against poisons.

The nourishment obtained through the gastrointestinal tract enters the blood via the liver. The liver is sorely taxed when acid wastes are constantly floating in the blood, and becomes life-threatening when the liver becomes congested with protein acid wastes.

Kidneys

Your kidneys are 75 to 80 percent water, and receive a full 20 percent of the cardiac output. Approximately one liter of blood per minute passes through your kidneys. Their primary duties are to keep the blood alkaline, and to extract acid. They remove acidic wastes such as uric acid, urea acid, and lactic acid, all of which must be dissolved in water.

When there's inadequate water, kidneys become over-stressed with too much acidity, and create kidney stones. Kidney stones are composed of waste acid cells and gummed together mineral salts, caught up in acid waste.

Increase alkaline water and reduce an intake of acid-forming foods to avoid the painful condition of kidney stones, and to prevent serious damage to the kidneys.

Spleen

Your spleen is 76 percent water, and has many supporting functions in the body. It's a filter for blood as part of the immune system. Old red blood cells are recycled in the spleen, and white blood cells and platelets are stored there. It also helps fight bacteria that cause pneumonia and meningitis.

Gallbladder

Your gallbladder is a small organ sort of "underneath" your liver. It stores the bile produced by the liver, an important role in the digestion of food, needed to digest fatty foods in the duodenum of the small intestine.

An erupted gallbladder is not only extremely painful, but life-threatening. Gallstones are the result of too much cholesterol, too much bilirubin, or not enough bile salts. Most readily available line of defense?: habitual intake of alkaline water.

Colon

The colon is made of muscle, and as such, is 76 percent water. It must be kept clean of accumulated acid wastes so it can perform its vital muscular action.

Excess acidic wastes collect on the colon walls, causing diarrhea or constipation. These wastes harden and are then reabsorbed into the bloodstream, inviting illness and disease. Regular, healthy bowel action indicates a healthy alkaline diet, and adequate alkaline water.

Bladder

The bladder is a muscular sac in the pelvis, about the size and shape of a pear.

Liquid waste, generated in the kidneys, travels down two tubes to the bladder, where it is stored. Layers of muscle tissue line the bladder, making it flexible to accommodate urine. The capacity of the bladder is approximately .85 to 1.3 pints (400 to 600 mL). Like the colon, the bladder needs a non-acidic environment to keep from becoming inflexible and less functional.

Your Precious Organs

The importance of water to every one of your organs cannot be over-stressed. Once again, my unflagging mantra: be well hydrated to support the health of every nook and cranny of your internal garden.

> *"The water cycle and the life cycle are one."*
> **Jacques Cousteau**

The Spine

The spine is made up of 24 bones, called vertebrae with ligaments and muscles connecting these bones together to form the spinal column. The spine gives the body form and function. Within the spinal column is the spinal cord, a bundle of nerves sending signals to the rest of the body.

There are three main sections to the spinal column: the cervical spine, the thoracic spine, and the lumbar spine. The first seven vertebrae form the cervical spine. The mid back, called the thoracic spine, has twelve vertebrae. The lower portion, the lumbar spine, is usually composed of five vertebrae, although some people have a sixth lumbar vertebra.

Cervical Spine (Neck)

The cervical spine is more mobile than both of the other spinal regions, allowing for neck mobility. There are also openings in each vertebra in the cervical spine for arteries to carry blood away from the heart and bring it to the brain.

Thoracic Spine (Mid Back)

The middle twelve vertebrae of the thoracic spine are connected to your ribs with narrow, thin intervertebral discs. Rib connections and smaller discs in the thoracic spine limit the amount of spinal movement in the mid back compared to the lumbar or cervical parts of the spine.

Lumbar Spine (Low Back)

The lumbar spine, called the sacrum, is a group of specialized vertebrae that connect the spine to the pelvis. The vertebrae in the lumbar spine area are the largest of the entire spine, and the lumbar spinal canal is also larger than in the cervical or thoracic parts of the spine, with more space for nerves to move about.

Intervertebral Disc

Intervertebral discs (discs between the vertebra) are 66-86 percent water. They cushion the vertebra from rubbing against each other, serving as shock absorbers.

Cerebrospinal fluid (CSF)

Cerebrospinal fluid is 99 percent alkaline water. It's a clear, colorless fluid in the brain and spinal cord, produced in the brain, and absorbed in the arachnoid granulations, small protrusions of the thin second layer that covers the brain, through to the thick outer layer of the brain.

There is 4.3 ounces (about 125mL) of cerebrospinal fluid at any one time, with nearly 17 ounces (500mL) generated every day. This fluid is constantly being reabsorbed, so that only 4.3 ounces is present at any one time. As it's 99 percent water, and 17 ounces is produced every day, it's obvious that water must be plentifully supplied

Cerebrospinal fluid is a cushion for the brain, providing it mechanical protection and immune protection. The cerebrospinal fluid is vital to cerebral blood flow.

Interestingly, there's a direct connection with cerebrospinal spinal fluid to the bony labyrinth of the inner ear via the perilymphatic duct in most people.

Cerebrospinal fluid pulses with the heart. (Check out the Wiki graphic to see this amazing beating brain: https://en.m.wikipedia.org/wiki/Cerebrospinal_fluid[1]).

Cerebrospinal fluid is derived from blood plasma and is similar to it, except it's nearly protein-free as compared with plasma, and has different electrolyte levels.

It is produced by the choroid plexus—a network of blood vessels in each ventricle of the brain—via an active process requiring the transport of sodium, potassium, and chloride, drawing water into the cerebrospinal fluid by osmotic pressure.

Carbonic anhydrase converts substances into bicarbonate and hydrogen ions, which are exchanged for sodium and chloride. Chloride, having a negative charge, moves with the positively charged sodium, to maintain electro-neutrality. Potassium and bicarbonate are then transported out of the cerebrospinal fluid.

Alleviating Back Pain

Seventy-five percent of your upper body weight is supported by the water volume that is stored in the spinal disc core, and the remaining 25 percent is supported by the fibrous materials around the disc. The spinal joints are dependent on the hydraulic properties of water, stored in the disc core. Back pain is frequently alleviated with adequate hydration.

Water Holds You Up

Fascinating! The bottom line is the profound importance of water for the part of your body that holds you up, your spine, with 99 percent water flowing through it. Keep those waters pure, clean, and electrically bio-available with fresh water.

Muscles

Your muscles are 76 percent water.

Do you ever get leg cramps in the middle of the night? Try drinking one or two glasses of warm/tepid water, straight down.

Why do we get those nasty leg cramps? According to the Mayo Clinic, they are most likely due to either strenuous exercise, or, conversely, lack of muscle use, and dehydration. The cramps are due to the muscles being triggered, but the action is stiff, not smooth.

A healthy muscle is shiny and strong, with elasticity and tension. Its expands and contracts like a big, wide, rubber band. When a shiny, healthy muscle is expanding and contracting, calmly going about its work, we take it entirely for granted. But a muscle that does not have what it needs to keep shiny and flexible is not able to do its work smoothly.

This difficulty registers to you as pain.

The tired, over-extended, thirsty muscle is calling out for the elixir that allows it to work and to run smoothly. All it wants, and all it needs, is to be watered.

Before, During, After Exercise

Drink one to two cups of water thirty minutes or so before exercise. This will help to ameliorate the impending fluid loss and provide fuel for your muscles during exercise.

Drink water during exercise to keep your muscles hydrated, shiny and flexible.
Drink plenty of alkaline water after exercise to replenish your muscles and your entire system with its much-needed fuel.

Is it not mysterious how we watch the gas gauge in our cars to make sure we don't run out of fuel on the way to and from the gym, but then not even pay attention to the "fuel gauge" of our entirely irreplaceable body? Be alert and attentive to your most important fuel gauge of all, and make sure your tank stays topped up.

Tones Muscles

Water is twelve times more resistant than air, so it takes more effort to move while submerged, according to Terry-Ann Gibson, Ph.D., associate professor of kinesiology at Boise State University. That means exercises in a pool are great muscle sculptors. Stand in water up to your neck and move your arms and legs as if you're cross-country skiing for a few minutes.

> *"Our bodies are molded rivers."*
> **Novalis**

Dem Bones – Osteoporosis

Your bones are 22 to 30 percent water.

Nobody argues that the body needs calcium to build bones, but many people do not know that bones are a complex matrix of numerous minerals, and if they are not all present, then strong bones cannot be built.

There are at least eighteen key bone-building nutrients essential for optimum bone health. The disconcerting truth is that it's easier to destroy bone through having excess acidity in the body than it is to rebuild bone. Adding to the dilemma is the ever-growing depletion of many trace minerals in farm soils. Our food grown on these soils contains less and less of the required nutrients.

Because many people's daily diet is significantly acidic, their bodies are leaching the calcium and alkaline stores from their bones in a desperate attempt to retain proper pH balance.

Healthy, alkaline water can help tremendously. Water lubricates the joints. The cartilage tissues found at the ends of long bones (shoulders, elbows, wrists, knees, ankles, hips) and the discs between the vertebrae of the spine hold a high volume of water, which lubricates movement.

When the cartilage has adequate water, friction damage in the joint is unlikely. But if the cartilage is dehydrated, the rate of abrasive damage is increased. This irritation, day in and day out, eventually results in joint deterioration and pain.

Even rheumatoid joint pain is frequently known to decrease with increased water intake, while flexing exercises bring more circulation to the joints.

Research shows that about 10-12 glasses of water a day significantly eases back pain and joint pain for up to 80 percent of sufferers[2].

When phosphoric acid or sulfuric acid manifests from the oxidation of nutrients that contain phosphorus and sulfur, these acids are too strong for the body to tolerate. It resorts to removing calcium from the skeleton to make phosphate or sulfate, a much weaker acid.

The urates and phosphate in kidney stones are the combination of acid and calcium, which is how osteoporosis develops. Taking calcium pills is inadequate because calcium, on its own, does not dissolve well.

Take your calcium with Vitamin D and magnesium, as they are catalysts for one another, and supplement all supplements with one or two glasses of water (unless taking your vitamin D, calcium, and magnesium in liquid form, which is highly recommended for superior absorption).

Collagen

There are 28 different kinds of collagen! Most collagen is in the range of 60-70 percent water. It's the main structural protein in the extracellular space in connective tissues in all animal bodies, and is 25-35 percent of your body's protein content.

The fibroblast is a cell in connective tissue that produces collagen, which is composed of amino acids that are wound together, forming triple-helices that produce long fibrils. Collagen is found predominately in tendons, ligaments, and our largest organ, the skin.

It ranges from being pliant, as in tendons, to its more rigid expression in cartilage, to the rigidity of bones.

Collagen is also found in plentiful amounts in your corneas, blood vessels, in your back's discs, in the gut, and in the dentin of your teeth. Your muscles are also one-to-two percent collagen, while six percent of your strong, tendinous muscles that attach your muscles to your bones is collagen.

Although there are 28 types of collagen, 90 percent of it is Type I, which is found in your skin, tendons, organs, bone, and blood vessels.

Here are the remaining main types of collagen[3]:

Type II: Cartilage

Type III: Reticulate, which forms a fine net-like structure, generally found with Type I collagen

Type IV: Forms the basal lamina, the base, thin layer or scale of organic tissue

Type V: The cell surfaces of hair and placenta.

Plenty of fresh water is needed for the ubiquitous nature of collagen, in all its forms, throughout your body. Having issues with your joints? Drink more alkaline water. Super-sore muscles after a strenuous workout or hard labor projects around the house? Your muscles are producing excess lactic acid. Help flush it out with water.

The inside and the outside of your hair and skin beg, and even demand to be nurtured and cleansed with alkaline water.

Skin
Water Keeps You Looking Young

"You can look significantly younger by keeping your skin hydrated," says Dr. Howard Murad, author of *The Water Secret: The Cellular Breakthrough to Look and Feel 10 Years Younger*[4], and associate clinical professor of medicine at the University of California, Los Angeles. "Water naturally plumps skin, fills in fine lines and wrinkles, and boosts a lackluster complexion."

Water helps to replenish skin tissues, moisturizes, and increases skin elasticity.

The Institute of Medicine's most recent water-intake guidelines suggest eleven 8-ounce glasses of water a day, and using products on the skin that contain hyaluronic acid, which creates a moisture barrier.

Complexion

Your face! Strangely enough, I can write about the effect of inadequate water on a person's insides, and many people will ignore it all. But mention how much plenty of alkaline water makes your face younger and more radiantly attractive, and people start to pay attention.

The cells in your face are not different from the cells in your blood, or your heart, or your intestines, in that they all need water. Water plumps up the cells of your face keeping it fresh and youthful.

The Bath

Allow your body's largest organ, your skin, to flush toxins in a bath of alkaline water. As mentioned before, pour in a cup of Epsom salts, which alkalizes the water with magnesium. As your body releases toxins in a relaxed, floating state, your skin absorbs much-needed magnesium.

You might also add bath oil to your blissful, rejuvenating time in the bath. Dr. Murad notes that bath oil attracts water to your skin and makes it smooth and silky, retaining the healthy hydration. However, I would first soak in the Epsom salts for awhile before adding bath oil so the magnesium can be fully absorbed by your skin.

Water Shrinks Pores

Soak a washcloth in steaming-hot water, then lay it over your face for a minute to open the pores. With the pores open, wash and rinse with warm water. Then splash your face repeatedly with cold water, which will shrink the pores. Makeup will look and stay smooth.

More Complexion Care

Drink warm lemon water first thing in the morning to reduce bacteria internally. This will also reduce breakouts. The warm lemon water has many other health benefits, as noted elsewhere in this book and in my book, *Save Your Life with the Phenomenal Lemon & Lime*[5].

Water Reduces Cellulite

Losing weight improves cellulite, but drinking water is the best way to plump skin, making the underlying fat cells less noticeable. Hydrating and losing weight by eating water-rich fruits and veggies also helps, and is healthy and tasty.

A study in Japan showed that women who got a lot of water from vegetables and fruits had smaller waists and lower BMIs than those who only drank their fluids. Fiber probably plays a major role in this instance.

Fiber and water are great friends, and are always happy to be linked together.

Water & Emotions & pH Balance

Your emotions affect your pH as much as what you eat and what you drink. Even, some evidence suggests, more. Your emotions have the profound ability to adjust your metabolic condition, making you more alkaline or more acidic.

AlkalineNationUSA.com[6] suggests that people with feelings that drive metabolic acids have more health concerns than people who have an acidic diet. As we can have control over both, why not become "Alkaline All the Way"? Alkaline foods. Alkaline water. Alkaline emotions.

Perhaps you're familiar with Bob Proctor's easy-to-remember, but much-abbreviated version of Gandhi's beautiful quote:

"Thoughts Become Things."
Bob Proctor

> *"Your beliefs become your thoughts,*
> *Your thoughts become your words,*
> *Your words become your actions,*
> *Your actions become your habits,*
> *Your habits become your values,*
> *Your values become your destiny."*
> **Mahatma Gandhi**

Thoughts, backed by energizing emotions, do move from (to quote one of my beloved teachers, Wayne Dyer) "No Where" to "Now Here."

Here's a thumbnail sketch of how that occurs. You have a thought, which requires energy, causing motion among your brain's cells to create that thought—you see how the thought has now, already, become "physical." The energy burned to create the thought produced acid. It's simply a fundamental, biological process.

But if the metabolic acids produced from thinking are not properly burned by an overall system that is slightly alkaline, the acids are moved out into the connective and fatty tissues. As discussed throughout this book, this causes a pH imbalance, which, if not brought into balance, leads to disease.

If the emotion attached to the thought is negative—fear, anger, guilt, depression, jealousy, shame, worry, frustration, and so forth—it produces more metabolic acids. The rate at which it does so depends on the length of time and the intensity of the emotion. When these metabolic acids accrue to a level that the body cannot keep up with dispelling them, the result is sickness, exhaustion, and weight gain.

But positive emotions—love, peace, belief, knowledge, happiness, flexibility, optimism, empowerment, etcetera—do not produce an overload of metabolic acids. The alkaline buffering works perfectly and in balance with your body.

You determine your emotions. First there's a thought, and, faster than lightning, you chose from your array of emotions which emotion you will attach to that thought. I know it's a perhaps somewhat mystifying concept at first if you've never contemplated this before.

We demonstrate our imperfect understanding of the thought-emotion paradigm when we say, "you made me angry." We all say it. But what's important to realize is that technically, we chose to be angry. We cannot be made angry.

Try it for yourself the next time you feel anger if you're resisting the idea. Determine to have another emotion, and refocus, reframe, and replace the anger with a less toxic emotion, or even an alkaline emotion. Frustration (less acidic) instead of anger. Observation, (slightly alkaline) instead of anger. And if you're going for the whole-healing winner, love (completely alkaline producing) instead of anger.

You will come to know the sensation of the acidic reaction, and, then feel the shift as the energy is removed from the choice of anger.

There's no future in anger! It only makes us sick, tired, and divided. It's not good for the individual. It's not good for the human family.

What is the one thing that helps support the ability to come to an alkaline calmness? Water. Water can almost instantly flush the negative emotion right out of your body. You have nothing to lose to drink a glass or two of alkaline water, while reframing the acidic emotion to an alkaline one. I know this will sound "woo-woo" to some of you. I only challenge you to try it. I welcome your comments about your experience.

Of course, it's helpful from the outset to plant positive thoughts in the garden of your mind so that they grow strong and are already well-established when called upon. You will learn that you can be, if you're not already, generally calm and joy-filled. This is a choice! I hope you make it.

Lots of water, lots of energizing and peace-centered, heart-mind, thought-emotions. Choose what you focus on. Choose how you interpret your life experience. Choose to keep it hydrated and smooth-running with brain-empowering water.

Water & Sleep
Water reduces body aches, cramped up muscles, pains in our feet, backs, necks, shoulders, and general overall discomfort.

Better Hydration Means Better Sleep
Drinking a glass of alkaline water before going to sleep helps the body accomplish its nightly repairs. Your body goes through a natural detoxifying process during sleep, and having fresh antioxidants at its disposal is not only essential, but contributes to a much more restful, rejuvenating, sleep.

I know many people don't want to have to get up in the middle of the night. But the healing benefit of adequate hydration during the over-night fast far outweighs stumbling into the bathroom and then back to bed.

Improve Your Sleep
Soaking in a hot bath of Epsom salts before bed can help you transition into a deeper, more restful sleep, a study at *Loughborough University*[7] found.

"The world turns softly
Not to spill its lakes and rivers
The water is held in its arms
And the sky is held in the water."
Hilda Conkling, Water

Water & DNA

DNA's double helix does not occur in isolation. Its entire surface is always covered by water molecules, which attach to the DNA with hydrogen bonds in a very specific way. However, the DNA does not bind all molecules in the same way. The texture of its hydration shell depends on the water content, while the water, in turn, influences the structure of the DNA.

Science News, May 25, 2017, reported that researchers at Cornell University used spectroscopy to observe a previously unknown characteristic of water—a chiral water superstructure surrounded the helical structure of DNA, which is itself chiral. (Chiral means an object or substance is not superimposable on its mirror image. For example, your left hand is not absolutely identical to the mirror image of your right hand.) This is an important discovery because most biomolecules and pharmaceuticals are chiral.

The upshot is that water plays a major role in DNA's structure and function. A broad range of behaviors of water structure in DNA's minor groove—where the backbones of the DNA's helical strand are close together—has been observed. This has profound implications in not only understanding the biological function of DNA, but is of tremendous import in research to discover new DNA-based materials, thanks to water.

Healing Crisis

What happens when you really change your lifestyle, get on a healthy diet, get enough rest, pause—really pause every now and then—and reset to be in the moment and drink enough healthy water?

What happens when you consciously choose to heal your body?

Remarkable things begin to happen—in your body, in your intellect, in your emotions. The innate wisdom of the body begins to reveal itself. When what comes into the body is of higher quality then the rubbish and the acidic animal flesh it has been compelled to work with, and when the water supply is adequate for the parched desert of your inner world, your body will diligently begin to cast off the inferior materials, and the fetid, stagnant water.

It will work energetically to manifest healthy blood, and build new, disease-free tissues.

Sounds wonderful, doesn't it? And it is! But what so many people are not prepared for—indeed, are not even aware of—is the impending healing crisis.

The body begins to jettison, through the clearing waterways of your internal streams and rivers, toxins such as caffeine and theobromine, removed from your tissues, put on a barge and hauled through your bloodstream to be carted off and eliminated. In the process of transportation, these toxins, these irritants, cause pain, headaches and other aches and pains, as well as feeling very tired.

After all, this is a great store of toxins being released and hauled through the body to be disposed of. In addition, removal of the toxins, many of which are stimulants, causes your heart to beat slower, which is good, but it feels, initially, like you're tired or depressed, because the rapid heartbeat in response to stimulants seems like exhilaration. It's not. It's your heart being burned up, used up.

This first aspect of the "healing crisis" will generally last about three days, as long as you stick with the clearing/cleaning, no matter how depressed you feel, no matter much the toxins you're removing from you body and life call to you.

After about three days for most people, this first wave of negative symptoms and depression abate. You suddenly feel stronger, brighter, lighter, more peaceful, Perhaps you have a sense of happiness for no particular reason. Always a good thing!

The Catabolic, Anabolic Processes

This first phase of the healing crisis is a catabolic process—large, defective molecules are being broken down by your enzymes into smaller components, and flushed out. The work of the body is to remove these inferior materials, and to make way for the healthy anabolic process, wherein the new molecules of nutritious food and plenty of healthy water are converted by enzymes into macromolecules, which are sent on their way to the healing process.

During this period most people lose weight, as stored fluids are flushed and stored fats begin to get cleared out. But then, as the healing body "gathers confidence" so to speak, that you're going to continue to provide plenty of water and first quality nutrients, it begins to dig deeper into the nooks and crannies and the backwaters of bad components. You will flow into another, deeper, level of healing.

You must stay the course, even though it's possible that you feel worse than in the first wave of "poison clearing." Regeneration is in process, please don't get in its way. Let your body heal. This period will last from ten days to as much as several weeks, depending on the intensity of regeneration and other factors of your unique self.

There is also a possibility that you'll sail through the healing without much sense of a downside, but it's not usual. So honor your body and yourself and engage in your healing mindfully, with patience.

Your essential energies in the periphery and external parts of your body—your muscles and skin—where you experienced healing in the first wave, now begin to move inward, once the muscles, and the organ of the skin, have been fortified. Your miraculously intelligent body begins to reconstruct your vital internal organs.

Diverting much of your essential energies, temporarily, deep into the internal areas of your body, produces a sense of weakness in your muscles. But in truth, you are becoming more powerful than you have been in a very long time. Maybe even since childhood.

Be patient with your healing. This is a critical time in the regeneration of your organs, deeper tissues, these deeper cells.

When you feel weak, sit quietly with the mental images of your organs rebuilding, picture old cells being cast out of your liver, your spleen, your lungs, your gallbladder, your kidneys, your intestines, your heart—all of your organs and tissues. Picture new cells, healthy cells, coming into place, making you healthier and stronger than perhaps ever before.

It may help to get an actual photograph or illustration of the internal organs, to concretely picture this process. However you honor the process of regeneration, this phase is crucial, and if you resort to any old habits; stimulants, depressants, being over-extended, poor diet, inadequate rest, inadequate water, you will interfere with the process of regeneration, and extend the healing process.

You're likely to observe that where you've tended to be the most "fragile" is where the most dramatic healing crisis occurs. If you have skin issues, as the skin contributes to the clearing, your skin will, for awhile, be more "eruptive." If you have a delicate digestive system, it will be more sensitive. If you're dealing with arthritis, your joints will likely become more painful. If you tend to headaches, the headaches will at first be worse.

You may be more susceptible to colds, flu, diarrhea, frequent urination. You may feel weak, tired, irritable, nervous, depressed. Clearing, clearing, clearing is what's going on! All of this has been lurking in your body, building up, waiting to turn into a life-compromising dis-ease.

Hang on! Love your body! It's so "grateful" now, to be able to cast off these poisons by the same route it has tried to "hide away" the poisons from your vital inner organs. It is arduously retracing, becoming more alive, more active.

You must have patience. Consider your body to be on sabbatical, and don't expect it to do its usual work when it's studying something new. Do not expect it to continue its usual work in the usual way. Rest and sleep more. Quietly rejoice as your feel crummier and crummier, knowing that the process is truly working, and that you are in the depths of a healing crisis.

And just when you feel your worst—weak, with various deep aches, perhaps never-before-felt pains—just when you're becoming alarmed that something worse must be going on, you'll suddenly move out of crisis. You'll feel strong, and healthy. But keep in mind, all these new cells, your regenerated tissues and organs, your healthy blood, are now in recuperation.

Your body is still using the bulk of its energies to shore up your deep, internal terrain. Continue to relax and recoup.

Retracing

What's happening during this time is the body is engaged in a process called "retracing." As it gets the sludge out of your arteries, veins, and capillaries, removes the excess bile out of your gallbladder and liver, removes the gassy, contaminated/contaminating brain-compromising masses, extracts the crippling, arthritic deposits in the joints, deletes the residuals of acidic drugs, excises the excess store of masses of fat—it is also "retracing" all of the patterns where those unhealthy cells were with new cells.

During this period, your weight tends to maintain as the amount of new tissue that is forming equals the amount of waste being replaced. After a period of replacing/retracing comes the third stage of anabolism, of building up the entire system.

There is sunlight at the end of the storm, so please ride it through. All these actions of your body are necessary. Don't try to minimize them or stay them with drugs. Drugs are acidic and will not contribute to the healing process.

Instead, indulge in sleep. Sleep is nature's number one healing process. Rest. Relax. Be calm. Be in the moment.

This healing process is an ongoing cycle of acceleration and plateau, acceleration and plateau. By that I mean you'll have a set of symptoms, you'll feel sick. You let the body flush out that set of toxins, and then you feel better. Then, another round of perhaps different symptoms, feeling sick, the next level of toxins are flushed out, and then you feel wonderful.

If you're dealing with a serious health issue, you may learn that somewhere in this healing process, the markers of the health concern have disappeared.*

All because you took the responsibility and power for your health into your own hands and replaced bad habits with calm, self-caring ones, replaced a bad, non-nutritive diet with a rich vegetable, fruit, grains, nuts, and seeds diet, replaced inadequate water with lots and lots of healthy, alkaline water.

You're now vitally alive and energetic, your skin looks fantastic, your eyes are bright and clear, your muscles are strong. You are calmer and more energetic than before the healing crisis. You've made it through your healing crisis and you're happy and healthy. And you'll stay that way, won't you? You'll keep your changed habits, superior diet, and adequate water, because you know you don't want to have to go through another healing crisis.

Life is rich when you're in good health!

*(None of these suggestions are meant to supplant or interfere with your continued relationship with your health care professional.)

> *"When you drink the water,*
> *Remember the spring."*
> **Chinese proverb**

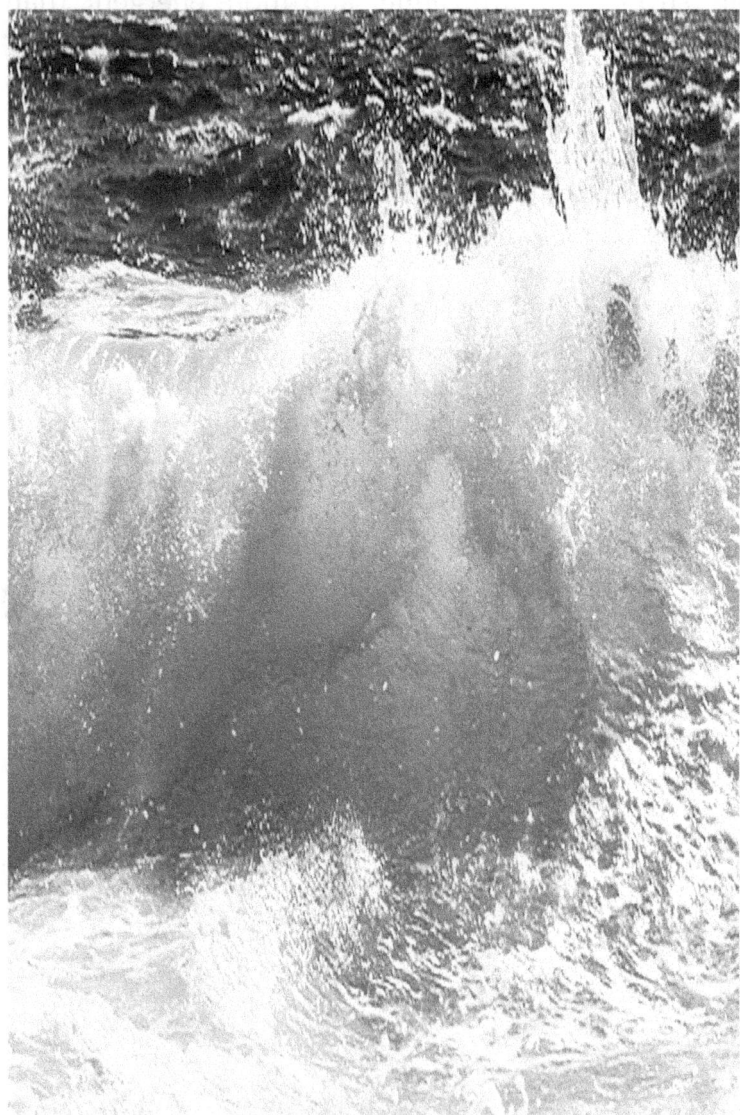

Chapter 3
Dis-Ease –
Water to the Rescue

All Dis-Ease

Quite a few health care professionals are arriving at the conclusion that diseases are caused by one central problem, which is the inability of the body to maintain a slightly alkaline pH balance, primarily driven by poor dietary choices and inadequate hydration.

Excess acid causes an imbalance that taps energy. The body's compromised and weakened energy cannot rid itself of excess acid, which, as previously mentioned, becomes systemic acidosis.

Acidic bacterium are found in arthritic joints, in arterial plaque, and in many other locations throughout the body. Cancer, heart disease, arthritis, osteoporosis, kidney stones, gallstones, tooth decay, etcetera, are all found in an environment of excess acidity. To prevent disease, or to manage a disease that has become established, acid imbalance needs to be overcome.

Sang Whang, author of *Reverse Aging*[1], wrote that all diseases are symptoms of the expulsion of acids from the blood and the tissues, and evolve from systemic acidosis.

Enervation—systemic weakness—prevents the elimination of acid waste-products. Retaining these metabolic acids in our organs and our tissues causes cellular disorganization and failed metabolism. We need only to rid the excessive acid waste-products from our bodies for our tissues and organs to be healthy.

Each organ presents its own particular symptoms, as any organ that is weakened below a minimal functional level from stress due to poor diet, poor habits, inadequate water, physical injury, work stress, personal life emotional stress—whatever the cause, is likely to become the location of the crises of systemic latent tissue acidosis. This gives rise to the idea that every organ has a unique and different disease.

The Cause of Disease—
Systemic Latent Tissue Acidosis

Sang Whang wrote: "The organ has nothing to do with cause, and directing treatment to the organ is compounding the problem. If prevention can be accomplished, then cures will not be needed!"

"When toxins accumulate beyond the toleration point, a crisis takes place. This we can call disease, but the only disease is systemic latent tissue acidosis, which will localize in the weakest parts of a body. What we call diseases are symptoms of the effects produced by forced elimination of acids through the mucous membrane.

"When this elimination takes place through the mucous membrane of the nose, it is called a cold. After years of this abuse, the mucous membrane thickens and ulcerates, the bones enlarge and close the passages. At this stage hay fever or asthma develops. When the throat and tonsils, or any of the respiratory passages become the seat of the crises of acidity, we have croup, tonsillitis, pharyngitis, laryngitis, bronchitis, asthma, pneumonia, etcetera.

"When the acids locate in the cranial cavity we have dementia, Parkinson's, Alzheimer's, muddled thinking, forgetfulness, and depression. When the acids locate in the gastrointestinal tract we have IBS, gastrointestinal dysmotility, autonomic dysfunction, carotid stenosis and ischemic colitis.

"When the acids locate in the pelvic tissue we have micro-calcifications of these acids that lead to tumors and cervical cancer or prostate cancer."

A simple translation: the retention of metabolic acids is the cause of all sickness and disease. The name the sickness or disease receives has to do with its location rather than its process.

Your Body —
A Homeostatic, Regenerating Mechanism
Your body has a homeostatic mechanism that must maintain a constant pH 7.365 in the blood, which works by depositing and withdrawing acid and alkaline minerals from various locations—bones, soft tissues, body fluids, saliva—as needed. In a healthy individual, this works beautifully, like clockwork, and bones and tissues are not compromised, but are regenerated.

Water is the Element that Makes
Your Body's System Work Beautifully

Sick Blood
Blood transports nutrients to every part of your body and cannot afford to be acidic. It needs to stay within a pH range that will maintain resistance to putrefaction and growth of malevolent organisms. The pH of blood must be 7.365. This is the ideal environment in which micro-organisms remain in symbiotic harmony with the body.

If the blood shifts the least little bit either way, these beneficial microforms die. Aggressive microforms that thrive in an acidic environment multiply and mutate into parasitic and pathogenic agents. Improper diet and inadequate water induces a proliferation of antagonistic microforms, which debilitate the body and cause death.

Every system in your body is used to support this slightly alkaline, correct, blood pH.

Blood cells have a negative charge on the outside and a positive charge inside, this is what keeps them healthy and magnetically repelling, keeping cells at a distance from one another, so the cells can flow. When your body is overly acidic, that acid strips your blood of its negative charge, and the blood cells no longer have the same repelling force. They begin to clump together.

When blood cells clump together, blood can no longer flow smoothly. It cannot get into all the little capillaries in your body to provide the necessary life-giving oxygen and nutrients. It can no longer give every cell the energy and rejuvenation it needs. This is one of the reasons why people wake up tired and unrested, needing more sleep. Their blood is not healthy, and is calling out for more water.

Water = pH Balance = Healthy Blood

Asthma
Histamine, which is a compound released by cells in response to allergic and inflammatory reactions causing contraction of smooth muscles and dilation of capillaries, plays a key role in regulating the way

the body uses and distributes water, helping to control the body's defense mechanisms.

In asthmatics, histamine increases when a person is dehydrated. The body's defense mechanism is to close down the airways. Asthma is frequently relieved when water intake is increased.

Cancer

Dr. Robert O. Young, along with Sang Whang and other doctors, believes that cancers are not a sickness or disease of themselves, but are symptoms of the build up of metabolic acids in the blood. When this happens, to maintain its required pH the blood throws the metabolic acids into the tissues. The accumulation of these acids significantly affects the ability of white blood cells to remove them, and the cells they are destroying, out of the body through normal elimination.

Dr. Young proposes that some cells change their makeup to survive in an acidic environment, and when they do, it's the beginning of cancer. Even if cancerous tumors are completely surgically removed, if the acidic conditions remain, new tumors are likely to develop in the same area.

Important for cancer treatment and prevention are the alkaline trace minerals rubidium, a rare soft silvery reactive alkali metal (chemical symbol: Rb), and cesium, a soft, silvery, extremely reactive metal, also belonging to the alkali metal group (chemical symbol: Cs).

Healthy Hydration

The University of Washington researched the connection between body hydration and diseases and detected a relationship between adults who habitually drank more than 5 glasses of alkaline water per day and a reduced risk of cancers. Bladder cancer was reduced 50 percent ("water dilutes the concentration of cancer-causing agents in the urine and shortens the time in which they are in contact with bladder lining"), breast cancer by 79 percent, and colon cancer by 35 percent.

Drinking alkaline water helps your body defray the build-up of metabolic acids. If these acids have the potential of supporting an environment in which cancer may develop, why not head it off before it even starts by keeping your internal environment slightly alkaline?

Diabetes

According to the International Diabetes Federation, 371 million people worldwide have diabetes, and according to the American Diabetes Association, 30.3 million Americans—almost ten percent—of the U.S. population has diabetes. Nearly 30 percent of seniors have diabetes. In addition, around 90 million Americans are prediabetic, which means that if they don't do anything to change their lifestyle, they will develop diabetes. Symptoms include increased thirst, frequent urination, blurred vision, and fatigue.

What is Prediabetes?

Prediabetes is a condition of inadequate production of the insulin hormone to move sugar out of the blood and into cells to fuel them as they make up tissues and muscles. As a result, sugars from food accumulate in the blood and the levels of sugar in the blood gets too high.

High blood sugar leads to kidney disease, blindness, amputations, heart disease, stroke, and high blood pressure.

Risk factors for prediabetes and diabetes include being overweight, being inactive, family history, inadequate or poor sleep, eating foods that contain cholesterol, and drinking cholesterol and/or sugar-containing beverages. Cholesterol is an animal product. There is no cholesterol in a plant-based diet.

Treating Prediabetes

In order to not become prediabetic or diabetic, a health-focused individual will increase physical activity, get adequate sleep, eat alkaline foods high in antioxidants, and drink alkaline water, while reducing or eliminating (yikes! I know) cholesterol and sugar-containing foods and beverages.

Dr. Theodore Baroody, author of *Alkalize or Die*[2], writes that the pancreas is highly dependent on an alkaline diet. When the pancreas has an alkaline diet, it is able to produce alkaline digestive enzymes and sodium bicarbonate, which it sends to your blood. Both the alkaline digestive enzymes and the sodium bicarbonate reduce the acidity in your body.

As discussed in the section on the stomach and intestines, your pancreas also regulates your blood sugar and helps give your body energy. Since diabetes is a disease where your body doesn't produce enough insulin to keep blood sugar in check, it is vital to keep your pancreas healthy. You can keep it happy with an alkaline diet and alkaline water.

Free Radicals = Oxidative Stress

It's possible that many people don't know that diabetes is largely caused by cellular deterioration. That's why you can fight diabetes with alkaline water. Not just because it's alkaline, but also, because it's full of antioxidants.

Cells deteriorate when they are attacked from the inside by excessive levels of acidic free radicals. The concentration of free radicals is measured as oxidative stress. So, to come full circle, when there are high levels of oxidative stress in your cells, your cells are damaged.

Alkaline water combats diabetes in two ways:

1. Provides the pancreas with the alkalinity it needs

3. Provides antioxidants that lower oxidative stress in the cells.

Water and Oxidative Stress

In a French study, participants who reported drinking more than 34 ounces of water a day had a 21 percent less chance of developing high blood sugar over the following nine years than those who reported drinking less than 16 ounces of water per day. (Dr. Ronan Roussel[3])

Supplementing Hydrogen-rich Water Improves Lipid & Glucose Metabolism in Type 2 Diabetes & Impaired Glucose Tolerance Patients

A Japanese study investigated the effect of ionized water on the oxidative stress associated with diabetes, hypertension, and atherosclerosis, on the premise that hydrogen has a reducing action.

The randomized, double-blind, placebo-controlled study specifically investigated the effects of hydrogen-rich water intake on lipid and glucose metabolism in 30 patients with type 2 diabetes, and six patients with impaired glucose tolerance. The patients had either 900 mL per day of hydrogen-rich water, or 900 mL per day of placebo water for eight weeks, with a 12-week washout period.

Several biomarkers for oxidative stress, insulin resistance, and glucose metabolism, assessed by an oral glucose tolerance test, were evaluated at baseline and at eight weeks.

The intake of hydrogen-rich water was associated with decreases in the levels of modified low-density lipoprotein (LDL) cholesterol by 15.5 percent, small, dense LDL by 5.7 percent, and urinary 8-isoprostanes (free radicals that result in cell damage) by 6.6 percent.

Hydrogen-rich water intake was also associated with decreased serum concentrations of oxidized LDL and free fatty acids, with increased plasma levels of the protein hormone, adiponectin (which regulates glucose levels and fatty acid breakdown), and the antioxidant, extracellular-superoxide dismutase. In four of six patients with impaired glucose tolerance, intake of hydrogen-rich water normalized the oral glucose tolerance test.

The results suggest that supplementation with hydrogen-rich water has a beneficial role in preventing or improving type 2 diabetes and insulin resistance. https://www.ncbi.nlm.nih.gov/pubmed/19083400[4]

In a German study[5], Type 2 diabetic patients who drank ionized alkaline water for four to six weeks noticed a drop in their blood sugar by an average of 25.7 percent. Type 1 diabetic patients noticed a drop of 33.3 percent over the same time period.

Other benefits appreciated by people drinking ionized water:

HbA1c levels lowered from 9.2 percent to 7.2 percent, reducing the risk of blindness by 45 percent in type 2 diabetic patients.

HbA1c levels dropped from 7.9 percent to 6.8 percent, again, lowering blindness risk by 45 percent in type 1 diabetic patients.

Type 2 diabetic patients reduced their medications by 47 percent, type 1 reduced their medications by 37 percent.

In both type 1 and type 2 diabetic patients, cholesterol, triglyseride, and LDL (bad) levels were reduced while HDL (good) levels increased.

Anti-Diabetic Effects of Electrolyzed Reduced Water in Diabetic Mice
This study examined the possible anti-diabetic effect of electrolyzed, reduced water in two different kinds of diabetic mice. (Electrolyzed water is discussed at length in Chapter 6.)

The study was based on insulin deficient type 1, and insulin resistant type 2 mice. Results were that the electrolyzed, reduced water provided as a drinking water significantly reduced the blood glucose concentration and improved glucose tolerance in both type 1 and type 2 diabetic mice.

The data suggest that electrolyzed, reduced water provides an orally effective anti-diabetic agent. Further studies on its precise mechanism are needed.
https://www.ncbi.nlm.nih.gov/pubmed/16945392[6]

Dr. Robert Young and Sang Whang note that where a person tends to accumulate solid acidic wastes in the body likely depend on their genetic makeup, suggesting, for example, that diabetes, itself, is not hereditary, but what is hereditary is the accumulation of solid acidic wastes around the pancreas. If the wastes are not given the opportunity to accumulate around the pancreas, diabetes has no environment in which to develop.

Arthritis

Joints affected by arthritis are the site of waste and toxin buildup due to the body fighting against its own auto-immune response system to heal damaged areas. Toxins are expelled by cells, and if we don't drink enough water, this waste remains at the joint, exacerbating symptoms and pain.

Symptoms are redness, warmth, swelling, and decreased range of motion in the affected joints. The onset might be gradual or quite sudden and shocking.

There are more than one-hundred types of arthritis! And, although they require different forms of treat-ment, in all cases it cannot hurt, and will, of course, help, to drink plenty of water.

Ankylosing Arthritis, Osteoarthritis, Rheumatoid Arthritis

Ankylosing arthritis of the spine, and osteoarthritis or rheumatoid arthritis in the back indicate water shortage in the spinal column and the discs, which are cushions composed of primarily water that support the weight of the body. Water is effective in treating these conditions by distributing electrolytes, which include potassium, sodium, bicarbonate, and chloride, around arthritic joints.

Electrolytes are not only soothing agents, they are essential for healthy cell development in arthritis affected joints, as well as the surrounding muscles and tissues, nourishing cells with nutrients.

Gout

Gout affects more than three million Americans. This condition and its complications occur more often in men, women after menopause, and people with kidney disease. Gout is strongly linked to obesity, hypertension (high blood pressure), hyperlipidemia (high cholesterol and triglycerides) and diabetes.

The first symptom of gout, which is a form of arthritis, is usually an episode of intense painful swelling in a single joint, most often in the feet, especially the big toe. The swollen site is usually warm to the touch and may be red. Fifty percent of first episodes occur in the big toe, but any joint can be involved.

The pain is from uric acid crystals that have settled in a joint or joints, causing stabbing pain, and is potentially disabling the joint. Pay attention to arthritis that comes and goes, which may indicate gout. Lifestyle changes include controlling weight, limiting alcohol intake, and adhering to a diet that avoids purines (which are most usually found in meats and fish). Purines break down into uric acid.

But the first line of defense to disable and wash out these stabbing crystals is to "water" them. Many people with gout also have minimal water intake. If you're dealing with gout, increase your water consumption. '(*Rheumatology.org*[7])

Uric acid is nearly insoluble in water, alcohol, or ether, undissolved due to low alkalinity in the blood. But it is soluble in solutions of alkaline salts, that is to say, alkaline water. Drinking alkaline water gradually elevates the blood pH. Gout has been shown to disappear, and arthritis to vastly improve, or disappear if damage is not too severe.

These & the Many Other Forms of Arthritis

The different forms of arthritis share in common inflammation of the joints. Water reduces inflammation, and alkaline water reduces inflammation faster. That's the bottom line on moving away from this debilitating pain. You cannot go wrong, and have nothing to lose, to drink more water. And may have much pain reduction, increased flexibility, and brightened mood to gain!

Obesity & Weight Loss

Why is there so much obesity in the world today?

Although the degree of starvation on Earth is appalling and unforgivable, Earth's current population is the first generation who will have more people die from being overweight than starvation.

Most people simply do not drink enough water. The curious result of this fact is that if your body is not getting enough water, you cannot tell when you are thirsty—you cannot tell when your body is begging for water. Thirst is mistaken for hunger, which leads to over-eating. Get in the habit of drinking a glass of water before your meals, and you'll see that it's easier to eat more mindfully. And to eat less!

> *Feel hungry, but want to weigh less?*
> *First drink down one, and better yet, two,*
> *glasses of water. Many of your "hunger*
> *signals" are actually thirst signals.*

In a University of Washington study, drinking one glass of water when feeling hungry stopped the hunger pangs in 98 percent of the dieters surveyed.

Renee Melton, MS, RD, LD, director of nutrition for Sensei, notes, "Many people find that if they have water before a meal, it's easier to eat more carefully." Getting healthy on a cellular level improves your life overall. When your body isn't over-exerting itself fighting toxins, you get better sleep, and, as I've mentioned previously, alkaline water helps you sleep better. Alkaline water also improves digestion of food so you get more energy from the food you eat.

With better sleep and better digestion of your nutrition, you'll feel less achy and less stressed. You'll make more thoughtful choices about what you eat throughout the day. You'll not be dependent on caffeine to give you a jump-start—which takes a toll. You'll be able to pause, reconsider, and pass on the candy bar, soda, or other sugar-laced habit.

Because your body feels better, you'll move more easily. You'll discover that you want to take walks and be physically active. All from simply drinking plenty of water!

Water & Metabolism
Being only one percent dehydrated causes a notable drop in metabolism. Meanwhile, clinical studies have shown that adequate hydration of your body:
1. has a dramatic positive effect on metabolism
2. improves the immune system
3. reduces joint and back pain
4. boosts energy
5. cuts down on hunger

"Your metabolism is a series of chemical reactions. Staying hydrated keeps those chemical reactions moving smoothly," observes Trent Nessler, PT, DPT, MPT, managing director of Baptist Sports Medicine in Nashville.

A primary reason for so much obesity in the world today is due to our bodies being besieged with an acid inner terrain. A body must work hard to remove toxic wastes, and it puts these toxins in fatty deposits as far away from the organs,especially the heart as possible, into the glutes, thighs, upper arms, and belly.

The body also pirates calcium from the bones and teeth, as the acidic diet does not provide enough alkaline minerals, calcium primary among them.

Dr. Robert O. Young points out that sugar is an acid and since the body must protect itself from the excess sugar we consume, it co-ops fat to encase the acid of sugar to protect the body from it.

Restricting water intake contributes to increased deposition of fat.

Water & Exercise
When embarking on a weight-loss plan, it may seem that the smartest thing to do is to start an active work-out program. But the recommendation from wise health-care practitioners is to start out gradually. Here's a bit of biology to back that up.

If we suddenly put the body to physical task beyond its present level, lactic acid builds up in the muscles and joints. Ironically, what your body will do with that lactic acid is create more fat to store it in. Thus, exercising too much is likely to add fat to the problem. The first line of approach, along with a step-wise ramping up of physical activity, is to make sure your body is healthier on the inside.

All of the toxins and fat that your body can't burn and use for energy must be put into storage. So your body creates fat cells to store it in. The best way to get rid of excess fat cells is to get rid of the acid and toxins stored inside the fat cells.

The more toxins that antioxidants neutralize inside your cells, the less your body needs to create new fat cells for storage, and the fat that is no longer needed melts away.

Water & Sodas

The dire health effects of soda are obesity in both adults and children. Two soft drinks—twenty-four ounces (two cans) is 20 teaspoons of sugar, 80 grams of sugar, 320 calories. This is more than three times the daily limit of sugar recommended by The World Health Organization (WHO), at a maximum of 25 grams of sugar per day. This is before even taking into consideration the other sources of daily sugar—breakfast cereals. Candy bars. Desserts.

What Happens when Drinking Soda?

Within the first few minutes of drinking a cola, ten teaspoons of refined, liquid sugar is zipping through your system. Again, this is the entire recommended amount of sugar for the day.

Soon, your blood sugar increases. In response, your body produces more insulin. Your liver encases the sugar in fat. At the same time, your body absorbs the caffeine from the cola, raising your blood pressure. This causes the liver to produce yet more sugar. The adrenaline high you experience, and become addicted to, is a response from your body, interpreting the sudden influx of sugar and caffeine as an attack. It's trying to protect itself.

In the process of eliminating these toxic elements from the bodily system, precious minerals exit along with the toxins, including calcium from your bones and teeth. Coming down from the absence of caffeine and sugar leaves a person irritable and tired. The response is to reach for another cola.

Don't do it! Drink water instead to repair and rejuvenate your body, reduce fat, save calcium, and do a million-and-one other beneficial goodies for your one-and-only body.

Water & Diet Soda

Have you ever noticed that most people who drink diet sodas are overweight?

This is because the chemistry of imitation sugars mimic the molecular structure of real sugar—but without any energy. Your metabolism, receiving the template for energy, but no energy arrives, "anxiously" awaits the energy. The instant any sugar comes along, it grabs onto it, in order to fulfill the false promise of the unreal sugar template.

So, in fact, "sugar free" is a deception. What it really is, is: "sugar-template-that-will-make-your-intelligent-body-try-to-fulfill-the-promise-it-was-given-by-saving-up-calories-in-the-fake-sugar-template."

Our poor, intelligent, bodies, ever faithfully trying to keep us alive, while we bask in our laziness!

Drink water instead. But if you must drink sodas, real sugar is a somewhat less awful poison than the fake sugar in so-called "diet sodas." Follow up a soda with water. A lot of water.

As mentioned elsewhere, a soda has a pH of 2.5, which is more than ten-thousand times more acidic than a glass of water at pH 7.4. I'll leave the math to you to determine how much water will counteract the poison of the soda.

Anorexia & Bulimia
Anorexia is when an individual all but stops eating. Bulimia is when a person regurgitates what they've

eaten. Both conditions are life-threatening and lead to electrolyte imbalance.

Although further discussion of these very serious conditions is beyond the scope of this book, it's important to understand that one of the first life-threatening aspects of anorexia and bulimia is the removal of electrolytes from the system. Alkaline water provides essential electrolytes.

Electrolytes are the minerals in your blood, critical to stay alive, and for muscle function. They include potassium, sodium, calcium, chloride, magnesium, and phosphorus, ions that carry a negative electrical charge. They are vital for maintaining the blood pH and for maintaining cell wall integrity. When electrolytes are inadequate, muscle weakness and severe muscle contractions are the result.

Individuals who seek help with these eating disorders are given electrolytes to work toward keeping their system in balance, and their bodies alive.

Shocking Obesity Rates of Children
Eighteen percent of children in the United States are obese. Most teens consume two to four soft drinks a day. A third of American children are consuming fast food once a day.

"Soft drink consumption in children poses a significant risk factor for impaired calcification of growing bones," Michael Murray, ND and Joseph Pizzorno, ND, wrote in the Encyclopedia of Natural Medicine.

This is the wide, fat, path to obesity, with children's bodies unable to handle the strain.

"... Billions of dollars are spent each year on fast-food advertising directed at kids," says Dr. David Ludwig, director of the obesity program at Children's Hospital in Boston.

Commercials show happy children eating toxic foods from their treasure boxes. These misleading advertisements affect what children grow up believing, and even hypnotize the parents into believing this product is good to feed their children.

While these companies try to promote fast food as "healthy," "healthy" and "fast food" shall forever remain an oxymoron. Tragically, the western diet has infected the world.

"We have truly a global epidemic ... affecting most countries in the world," said Dr. Philip James, chairman of the International Obesity Task Force, predicting a massive weight gain in children around the world. "(Children) are being bombarded to eat all the wrong foods. The Western world's food industries have precipitated an epidemic with enormous health consequences."

For the Better Health of Children

The obesity among children will not only shorten their lives, but, of course, will lead to a continuing unhealthy lifestyle when they reach adulthood, sadness for individuals, and a huge poor-health burden on society.

If everyone was to do one, single, thing to contribute significantly to the future of our children, it is to cut out soda, sugar-laced juice boxes, and all high sugar drinks, replacing them with pure, simple, alkalized water. Children follow the example they are given. Parents need to be parental, and set the example by drinking lots of water, cutting out the sugar.

Studies have shown that children who are given water to drink as children keep this habit into adulthood. Study not needed. It's obvious and not under the heading of "rocket science" that childhood habits continue into adulthood.

Water Helps You Lose Weight

Drinking water contributes to weight loss by helping flush out the by-products of fat breakdown.

A study at the National Meeting of the American Chemical Society reported that adults who drank two 8-ounce glasses of water before breakfast, lunch, and dinner ate fewer calories during each meal.

Over the three months of the study, participants in the water-drinking group lost an average of five pounds more than dieters who didn't drink two glasses of water before meals, proving that it's an effective appetite suppressant.

DRINK WATER TO LOSE WEIGHT

A Short Miscellaneous List of Water Positives
Lowers Stress
"Water's calming effects are immeasurable," says Gabrielle Bernstein. "The sound of running water triggers a soothing response, which can reduce stress … feng shui emphasizes the benefits of the sound of running water … to enhance overall happiness and peace."

Beautiful Skin
Acidic water at 5.5 pH is considered beauty water in Japan. It's a natural astringent, much healthier for skin than chemically-based astringents.

Shiny Hair
A cool-water rinse leaves hair glossier. The chilly water constricts the cuticle layer of hair so it lies flatter, making strands smoother and more reflective.

Water & Sore Throat, Headache, & Back Ache

The Mayo Clinic recommends a saltwater gargle the next time you feel a sore throat coming on. Stir one-quarter teaspoon of, preferably, sea salt into an eight-ounce glass of warm water. Sip, and gargle.

Water also helps relieve headache and back pains due to dehydration, a common reason for headache.

Cleans Naturally

When water is combined with other natural ingredients it becomes a fantastic cleaning agent.

Here are tried-and-true cleaners from Sara Snow's Fresh Living:

Scrub: Make a paste of water with baking soda for a tub and sink scrub.

Disinfect: Mix equal parts water and distilled white vinegar in a spray bottle to disinfect kids' toys, cutting boards, kitchen counters, etcetera.

Glass Cleaner: One-quarter cup lemon juice in a spray bottle filled with water.

Strong Alkaline Water

A water ionizer that can make strong alkaline water eliminates the need to purchase household bleach (pH 12.6) or ammonia (pH 11.5). If you produce an alkaline water at these pH levels, it replaces earth-harmful and expensive products.

Strong Acidic Water

At the same time, soaking sponges and toothbrushes in ionized water with a pH below 4 keeps them sterile.

"Gardens dream about water."
Michael P. Garofalo, Pulling Onions

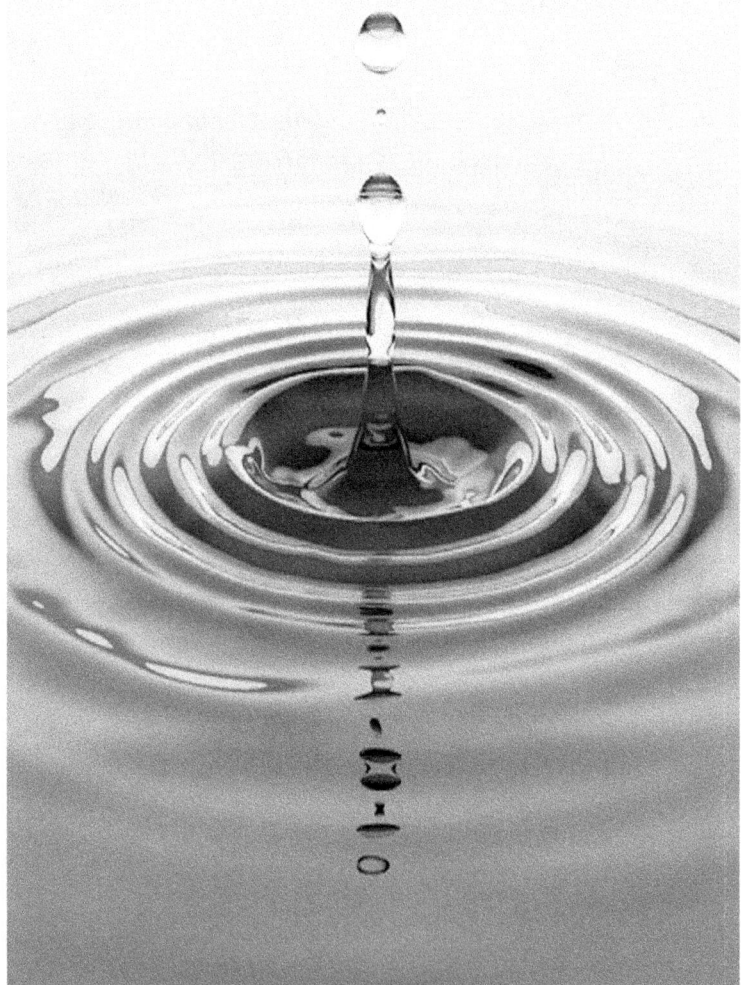

Chapter 4
Water & pH Balance

The pH of Water, Why is it Important?

*T*he measure of pH in water is extremely important. Water must be very nearly neutral or slightly alkaline in order to support life. pH testing measures how acidic or basic (alkaline) any substance is. The pH scale ranges from 1 to 14, with 7 being neither acid nor alkaline, referred to as neutral. Any measure of pH that is below 7 is acidic, a measure above 7 is base or alkaline.

Understanding the Range of Acid to Base

To get a clearer picture regarding the pH in water, it can be helpful to know the pH of other substances. For example, battery acid has a pH of one, which is the extreme of acidic. At the other end of the scale are substances such as lye and ammonia, which measure in the 13-14 pH range, and are extremely alkaline.

How the pH Scale Works

The pH in water is readily affected by chemicals that may be found in water. Therefore, testing the pH of water is an excellent way to learn about the health of a given environment. The pH scale is logarithmic—each number is ten times more or 10 times less acidic than the next higher or lower whole number. Water with a pH of 6 is ten times more acidic than water with a neutral pH reading of 7.

pH 8 is 10 times more alkaline than pH 7
pH 9 is 100 times more alkaline than pH 7
pH 10 is 1,000 times more alkaline than pH 7
pH 11 is 10,000 times more alkaline than pH 7
pH 12 is 100,000 times more alkaline than pH 7
etcetera
or, conversely,
pH 6 is 10 times more acidic than pH 7
pH 5 is 100 times more acidic than pH 7
pH 4 is 1,000 times more acidic than pH 7
pH 3 is 10,000 times more acidic than pH 7
pH 2 is 100,000 times more acidic than pH 7
etcetera

As mentioned elsewhere, a cola has a pH of 2.5, meaning it is nearly 100,000 times more acid than your blood at pH 7.4.

pH Acidic Water

The importance of measuring the pH in water is that this reading determines the biological availability of healthy nutrients in the water, such as carbon and nitrogen, and the measure of toxic heavy metals, such as copper and lead. These components either contribute to sustaining, or contribute to damaging, life. At a lower pH reading toward acidic, metals become more soluble and therefore more toxic. There is an unpleasant metallic taste to the water.

Concern and Cure for Acidic Water

In the U.S., much tap water, and even some well water, depending on location, is so penetrated by toxic bacteria thriving in acidic water and environmental and industrial pollution in the form of heavy metals and chemicals, that it is not safe for drinking.

Currently, U.S. city water, wells, rivers, and lakes adjacent to cities, are contaminated and acidic. A water filtration system in the home that can remove over 90 percent of the contamination in your water system is a wise measure. In addition, this alkaline, healthy water goes out into the ground water, doing more good than harm to all water.

> *"Nature is blamed for failings that are Man's,*
> *And well-run rivers have to change their plans."*
> **Sir Alan Herbert, Water**

pH Testing Your Water

There are a wide range of methods to test your water from very inexpensive pH testing strips, to extremely affordable home testing kits that test for lead, bacteria, pesticides, iron, copper, chlorine, nitrates, nitrites and pH, to sending out your water to a lab for more detailed information, but considerably more expensive.

The ten-test kit seems like an excellent choice. If all these tests are in a normal range, you need not test further, unless you have a particular concern. You can often get pH strips at your corner drugstore. They are great to test both your household water, and your own bodily pH. Not extremely sophisticated, but adequate to determine basic information. Again, if the strips show a normal, healthy range, there is no need to go further. If they show an extreme of acidity for either your water or yourself, then further action is advised.

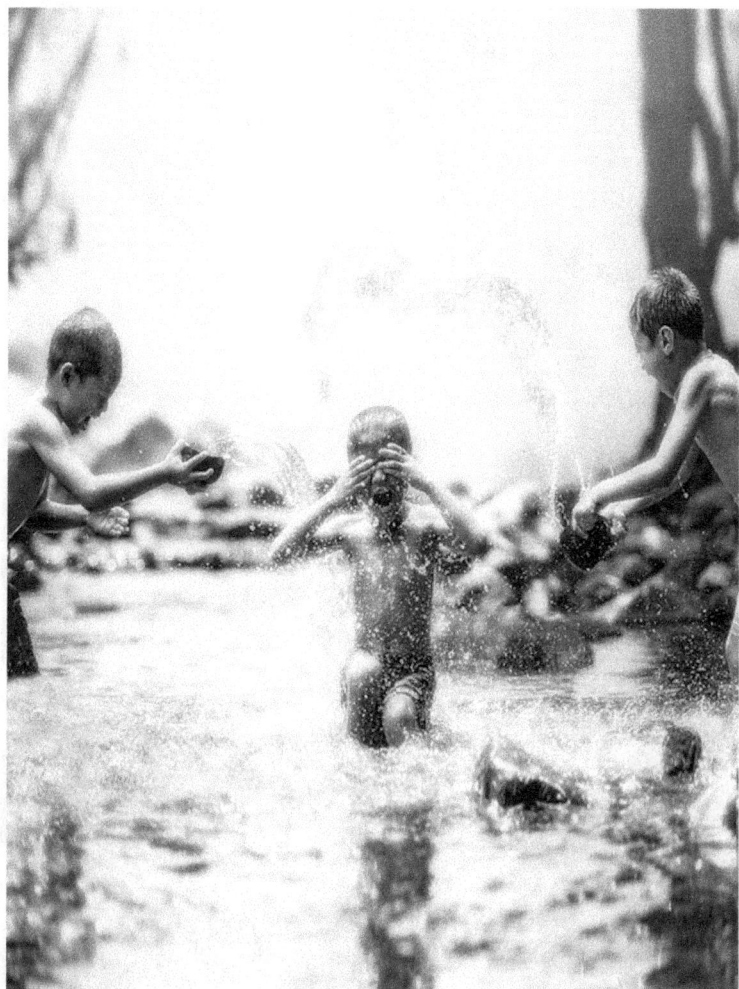

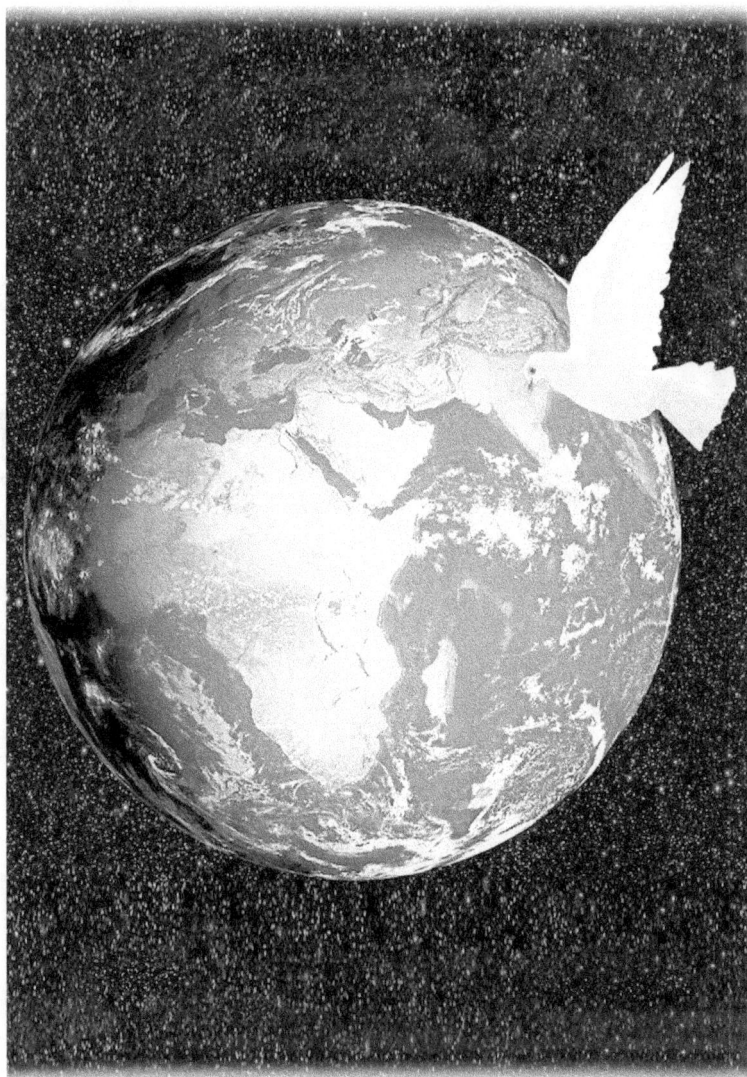

Chapter 5
Sick Water

*"When we try to pick out anything by itself,
we find that it is bound fast by a thousand
invisible cords that cannot be broken
to everything in the Universe."*
John Muir

*B*efore the industrial revolution, we drank water from natural sources—rivers, streams, lakes, the ocean. This "living water" is enriched by sunlight and is full of antioxidants.

But people living in cities no longer have water that comes directly from natural sources. The water that comes out of the tap has been pumped from rivers and lakes to giant metal holding tanks where it sits, unmoving, while the metal of the tank leaches into the water.

In that static condition the ions dissipate, and there's no longer any antioxidants in the water. At the same time, your municipal government assures that fluoride and chlorine are in the water, along with the metal contaminant.

Water Poisons

There are a disconcerting number of poisonous substances in our water, our household water. In the year 2,000, there were listed eight thousand chemicals in U.S. household water. The EPA (Environmental Protection Agency) is monitoring them—I'm not too sure what that means in pragmatic terms.

Here's a tiny window into some of the dangerous chemistry in our water:

Chromium-6: Confirmed cancer-causing chemical

Chlorine: Is added to all US municipal water supplies, supposedly to disinfect the water. Do you find the resultant wide-ranging effects acceptable? Namely: hardened arteries, destroyed bodily proteins, irritated eyes, irritated skin, irritated sinuses, aggravated allergies, skin rashes, psoriasis, eczema, emphysema, asthma and other respiratory problems, and increases in the risk of miscarriage.

Chloroform: Chloroform is a by-product of chlorination, and causes the proliferation of free radicals.

This leads to accelerated aging, causes normal cells to mutate, and causes cholesterol to oxidize. It is a confirmed carcinogen.

DCA (Dichloro acetic acid): Another chlorine byproduct, it also affects cholesterol metabolism, and has caused liver cancer in lab animals.

MX (Chlorinated acid): MX has been found in all chlorinated water. It's known to cause genetic mutations and cancer. It has been proven to cause bladder and rectal cancer.

Found in 33 states:
Polyfluoroalkyl: Confirmed cancer-causing chemical, and is hormone disrupting,
and
Perfluoroalkyl: Confirmed cancer-causing chemical, also hormone disrupting.

According to extensive research, chlorinated water is the cause of nine percent of all bladder cancers and 15 percent of all rectal cancers in the US! When are we going to wake up?

When you take a warm shower, your pores open, so not only are you inhaling the chlorine vapors, you are absorbing chlorine through your skin into your blood-stream. The receptive organ of your skin absorbs more chlorine during a ten-minute shower than when you drink eight glasses of the same water.

It's possible to evaporate chlorine and kill some micro-organisms by boiling water. However, other chemicals and all the dissolved solids remain, along with endotoxins from the boiled bacteria. These endotoxins can generate pyrogens, a substance typically produced by a bacterium, causing fevers when released into the blood. Pyrogens are more harmful than the live bacteria they replace.

Phthalates have been found in tap water. Phthalates are used for making plastic. In addition to phthalates there is chlorine, fluoride, chloramine (ammonia and chlorine combined), pharmaceutical drugs, nitrates and nitrites from farms, cleaning agents, chemicals from household products, heavy metals like arsenic, lead, and mercury.

The lead in tap water causes learning disorders in children. Also, outbreaks of waterborne diseases can be linked to drinking water.

Bottled Water
Even though bottled water has become popular, it's now fairly common knowledge that it has its own set of issues, the central one being one that it shares with tap water—when water sits, unmoving, the alkaline properties dissipate, and the water becomes acidic, in addition to the fact that chemicals are leaching from the plastic into the water.

A Suffolk County, New York, study tested 88 bottled waters and discovered benzene, Freon, kerosene, toluene, trichloroethylene, and xylene. A study by the National Resources Defense Council (NRDC) found that one-fifth of the sampled bottled waters contained neurotoxins and carcinogens including styrene, toluene and xylene.

Another NRDC study found that, out of 103 brands of bottled water, one-third contained traces of arsenic and E. coli. A popular brand of U.S. water was forced to announce a world wide recall when an unsafe level of benzene was found in their bottled water.

You may be surprised to learn that bottled water is not regulated like tap water is. In fact, unlike tap water, it's one of the world's least-regulated industries. Regulations allow bottled water to contain some contamination by E. coli or fecal coliform, and don't require disinfection for cryptosporidium or giardia. These are parasites. Do you really want harmful parasites living in you or your children?

It's shocking to discover that bottled water can be, and likely is, contaminated and yet still sold in the U.S. As tap water is a public resource, extensive documentation on its quality and content is made available to the populace. But there's not the same accountability for bottled water, regulated like a soft drink, rather than a public resource.

Regardless of springs, mountains, and other bucolic scenes on the labels, bottled water is often simply tap water, NRDC and Consumer Reports have found.

One very popular and prevalent brand of water is drawn from the municipal water supplies of Detroit, Fresno, and other cities. Coke and Pepsi, who are the main producers of bottled water under different brand names, also use tap, not spring, water.

All India Institute of Hygiene and Public Health found cadmium, chromium, lead, antimony, and DEHP in Pepsi, Coca-Cola, Sprite, Mountain Dew, and 7-UP. All were packaged in polyethylene terephthalate— PET bottles.

Another American team in Pennsylvania analyzed 37 brands of bottled water, 28 of them from Europe, for alkalinity, aluminum, barium, beryllium, boron, cadmium, calcium, chloride, chromium, cobalt, copper, fluoride, iron, lead, lithium, magnesium, manganese, mercury, molybdenum, nickel, nitrate, pH, phosphate, potassium, silver, sodium, specific conductance, sulphate, tin, vanadium and zinc. Twenty-four of the 37 did not comply with drinking water standards of the U.S.

With the exception of Mountain Valley, a United States water, every one of them failed to pass EEC or WHO limits on one or more counts.

When you factor in the devastating environmental costs associated with bottling a public, natural resource, the difference between bottled and tap becomes even more dramatic.

The most common plastic used in water bottle manufacturing is PET (polyethylene terephthalate), an environmentally unfriendly substance. It requires nearly 5 gallons (17.5 kilograms) of water to produce one quart (one kilogram) of PET plastic. Mind boggling. Several times as much water is used to make PET bottles than is put into them.

The production of PET plastic also produces numerous byproducts that are extremely harmful to the environment. *Statistic Brain* (StatisticBrain.com) reports that 35 billion bottles of water are sold annually in the U.S., yet not even ten percent of these bottles are recycled. Over 90 percent end up in the trash.

That's 31.5 billion plastic bottles in landfills—bottles that require a ridiculous amount of water to produce, that contaminate our environment to produce, that leach poisons into the water you will drink, that contains water, ready-made with its own poisons, less healthy than tap water.

Thirteen billion dollars is spent in the U.S. annually on bottled water, and 75 billion dollars is spent annually on bottled water, world wide.

Go. Figure.

Purified Water
More bad news about bottled water: most bottled waters are purified water, and purified means everything has been stripped from the water.

The same is true of water that has been distilled or filtered through reverse osmosis. It has had the oxygen, and the alkaline minerals—the antioxidants— removed. It's in an acidic state. Be aware that when a bottled water is labeled as a vitamin water, it is still acidic. When water has no minerals and is acidic, it is actively absorbing substances out of your body.

Purified water is fine for cleaning lab equipment, or watering plants, which thrive on acidic water. But it's not fine for the human body. The more acidic your water (and remember, it should not be acid at all, but alkaline) the more it steals minerals and nutrients from your body, including the calcium from your bones and teeth, and the magnesium from your entire system, the more you will feel— and be—dehydrated.

Distillation is a process of boiling water to evaporation, then condensing the vapor. Reverse osmosis or purified water is free of dissolved minerals. Do not fast and drink purified water, as you'll experience a rapid loss of your precious electrolytes, including: sodium, potassium, chloride, and essential minerals, such as your all-important magnesium. These deficiencies are life-threatening and lead to health issues including irregular heart beat and high blood pressure.

Cooking foods in distilled water pulls minerals out of your food. Not good!

When purified water comes in contact with air it absorbs carbon dioxide, making it acidic. The more purified water you drink, the higher your body acidity will become. Acidic, purified water can dissolve metals.

Soft drinks are made from purified water. Soft drinks pull huge amounts of vital calcium, magnesium, and other trace minerals from your body, pouring them into the urine and exiting your body. This mineral loss drives osteoporosis, osteoarthritis, hypothyroidism, coronary artery disease, high blood pressure, and a number of other diseases that cause premature aging.

Bacteria & Heavy Metals in Household Tap Water

Many water pipes beneath cities are old and corroding and may be carrying dangerous and drug resistant bacteria such as legionella, mycobacteria, and pseudomonas. Corroding pipes also deposit lead and other heavy metals in the water, which are carcinogens. Heavy metals increase oxidative stress in our cells, making us more susceptible to illness and disease.

According to the EPA, only nine states report safe levels of lead in the water: Alabama, Arkansas, Hawaii, Kentucky, Mississippi, Nevada, North Dakota, South Dakota and Tennessee.

Acid Rain

Acid rain is rain, snow, fog, or other precipitation that is full of acids which collect in the atmosphere due mostly to burning fossil fuels such as coal, petroleum, and gasoline. Rain is a source of sulphuric acid, lead from petrol and diesel fumes, sulphur dioxide, carbon monoxide, and benzine derivatives from industry.

Sulfur and nitrogen oxides in the atmosphere form compounds that are transported long distances, and subsequently deposited on Earth's surface in both wet and dry forms.

Although the term "acid rain" is widely used, the dry deposit of acidic compounds account for 20 to 60 percent of the pollution deposits, in both particle and in gaseous forms. Acid rain is more accurately named "acid deposition." Both local and distant emissions contribute to atmospheric acid deposition.

This acid deposition acidifies lakes, streams, coastal waters, and large river basins, causing soil nutrient depletion, decline of forests, and agricultural crop damage, with a severe negative impact on ecosystem biodiversity.

"In an age when man has forgotten his origins and is blind even to the essential needs for survival, water, along with other resources has become the victim of his indifference."
Rachel Carson

The World's Fresh Water—in Crisis
Toxic Chemicals are Destroying Groundwater The World Over

The following bullet points are noted by the Worldwatch Institute:

• Toxic chemicals contaminate groundwater on every inhabited continent, endangering the world's valuable supplies of freshwater. Pesticides, nitrogen fertilizers, industrial chemicals, and heavy metals are found in groundwater everywhere.

• Twenty-eight percent of the groundwater in the Netherlands used for drinking contained perchlorate, a dry cleaning solvent.

• The U.S. Environmental Protection Agency (EPA) notes that over 100,000 gasoline storage tanks are leaking chemicals into groundwater.

• About 97 percent of the planet's liquid freshwater is stored in underground aquifers.

• Waste disposal sites leak liquid wastes into groundwater. Nearly one-third of all humanity relies almost exclusively on groundwater for drinking.

• Over half of the U.S. population, and 99 percent of its rural population is dependent on groundwater. And yet, every state has contaminated groundwater.

• About 70 percent of the world's freshwater goes to irrigation. In the U.S., 70 percent of the crop goes to feed livestock instead of humans. Meanwhile, livestock produces ten times the waste that the human population produces, contaminating our groundwater ten times faster.

• Current U.S. Environmental Protection Agency (EPA) information on US pesticide usage reports that over two billion pounds of pesticides are used in the U.S. every year. This is 22 percent of the estimated 5.2 billion pounds of pesticides used worldwide (while the U.S. population is 4.4 percent of the world's population). Runoff from fertilized fields and industry contaminates our household water.

• Groundwater replenishes rivers, streams and wetlands, providing much of the flow for the Mississippi, the Niger, the Yangtze and many other human-survival rivers. Some of these rivers will cease to flow year round if their groundwater supply continues to be compromised.

• India's Central Pollution Control Board found that groundwater was unfit for drinking in all 22 major industrial zones it surveyed in 1997-1999.

• 80 percent of India's villagers depend on groundwater for drinking.

• More than half of groundwater sampled contained nitrate at levels above safe limits in Mexico's Yucatán Peninsula.

• Gasoline and other contaminates leak from underground storage tanks. Pollutants and disease seep from poorly constructed landfill systems. Nine billion gallons per year of the most hazardous liquid waste in the United States—solvents, heavy metals and radioactive materials—are injected directly into groundwater via thousands of injection wells.

• Since 1943, billions of gallons of radioactive wastes have been dumped into soils and aquifers in Washington State by the Department of Energy's Hanford Nuclear Reservation. Some of this waste has a half-life of 250,000 years.

June 8, 2017 - EPA: Radioactive Waste Still Flooding Columbia River:

KENNEWICK, Washington – Groundwater contaminated with radioactive waste; hexavalent chromium and strontium-90, is still flowing into the Columbia River from the decommissioned Hanford nuclear facility in Washington State.

Added to the list are the threats and dangers to Earth's oceans and seas. These issues are so vast, that it is a book of its own. But for the present purposes, here's a mere "tip of the iceberg." Thanks to Boat International (boatinternational.com) for the following points:

• Pollution: Major oil spills, dumping of toxic and radioactive materials, absorption of about half of the CO_2 created by burning fossil fuels.

• Plastic debris: It's really out of control. On one Cornish beach, a group of concerned citizens picked up nearly 600,000 pieces of plastic.

• Illegal, unreported and unregulated fishing: pirate fishing causing losses to coastal areas of up to 23 billion dollars annually. Illegal fishing is as much as 40 percent of the catch in some fisheries.

• Fishing coral reefs: coral reefs cover less than one-quarter of one percent (.025%) of the world's oceans, but are the home of fully one-quarter (25%) of all marine life, with up to two million species. More than half of the resident fish have disappeared from most coral reefs.

• Acidification: The pH of the seas has been the same for 60 million years, and now it is becoming acid due to the buildup of carbon dioxide.

• Melting ice caps: average temperatures in the Arctic are rising twice as fast as they are elsewhere in the world. An obvious hardship for the resident creatures.

- Natural, wild areas have become endangered, as nothing is remote anymore.

- And a new threat: deep sea mining.

Plus the following from Marinebio.org (please go to their site to see amazing videos and to learn more):

- The populations of many ocean species are decreasing at an unsustainable rate. The number of marine life species listed as endangered includes: whales, dolphins, manatees, dugongs, salmon, seabirds, sea turtles and sharks, to list only a few, with disappearing species on the rise.

This species extinction is due to loss of habitat, spread of disease, pollution, and illegal fishing practices.

*"The frog does not drink up
the pond in which he lives."*
Native American Saying

Is There Any Promise for the Future?
Not to leave this array of beyond-dismaying facts with only bleak and depressing information, there are people who are employing their brilliance and creativity, willing to think in constructive and inventive ways to help our little planet heal from our willful and destructive behavior, destroying the planet's water.

Here are a few examples of pollution solutions:

• Since 1998, all the farmers in China's Yunnan Province have eliminated their use of fungicides, while doubling rice yields by planting more diverse varieties of the grain.

• Water utilities in Germany pay farmers to switch to organic operations because it costs less than removing farm chemicals from water supplies.

• Manufacturers can reduce groundwater pollution by reusing materials and chemicals, keeping them out of landfills, and reducing leakage from landfills. Companies are building "industrial symbiosis" parks in which the unusable wastes from one company can be used by another.

• In Sweden, where chlorinated solvents were phased out, companies report economic advantage in switching to water-based solvents derived from biochemical sources such as citrus fruits, corn, soybeans, and lactic acid.

• Pollution taxes in the Netherlands helped the country slash discharges of mercury, arsenic, and other heavy metals into waterways by up to 99 percent.

• This is your bullet point—what are you changing in your life to contribute to healing Earth's waters?

"Don't let this time, the time you live in,
be the darkest of all dark ages
to future generations.
Do your part to bring Earth,
her land, her oceans, and her creatures,
back to health...."
Blythe Ayne, Ph.D.

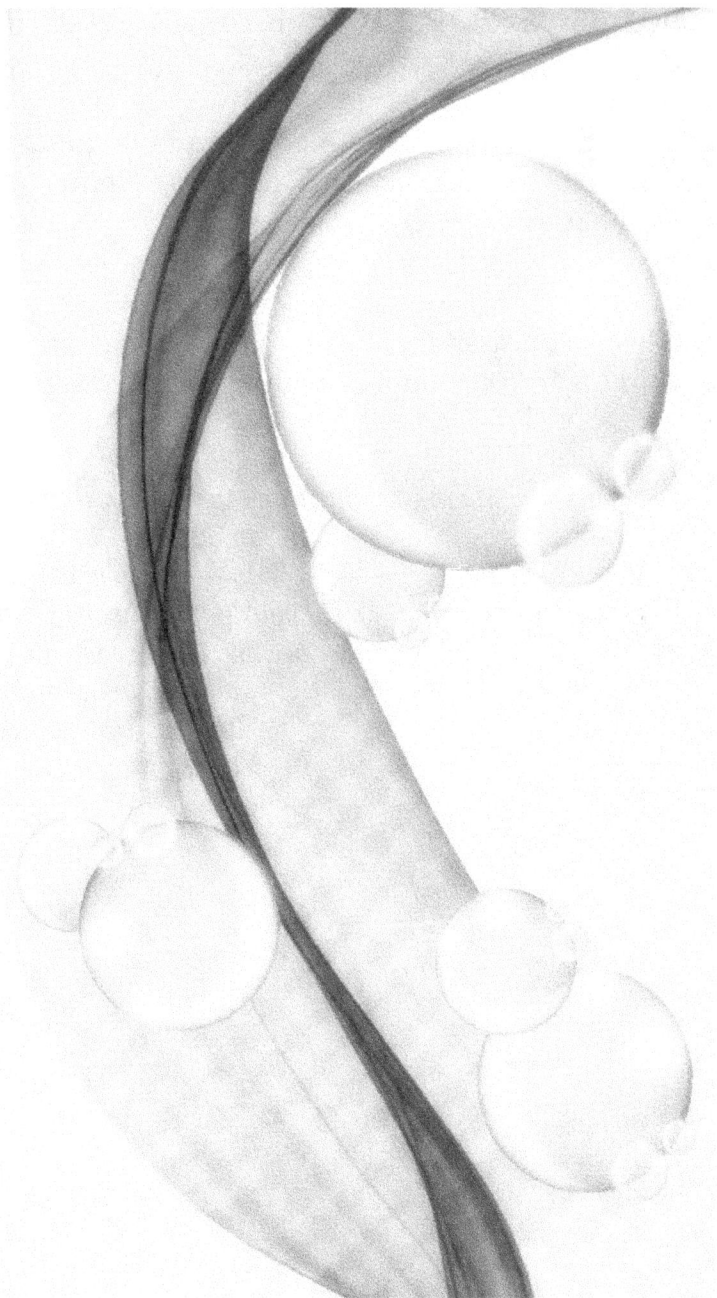

Chapter 6
Ionized Water, Electrolyzed Water, Hydrogenized Water, Gel Water

Alkalized, Hydrogenized Water

*I*onized water is electrolyzed water, and electrolyzed water is water that has been energized by the process of water electrolysis, producing the antioxidants that contribute so significantly to your health.

Ionized water donates electrons to "active oxygen"— also known as free radicals. No longer active, but instead, stable, this oxygen doesn't need to steal ions from your normal, healthy molecules. Free radicals do steal ions from your healthy molecules, rendering them unstable and prone to the invasion and aggression of diseases, pain, weakness, aging.

How is Water Electrolyzed?

Water ionization is what happens to the water molecule after it passes through water electrolysis. Electrolysis is produced either by the sun energizing the water, or the water rushing over rocks (or both processes), or by electricity passing through plates inside a water ionizer, converting the H2O water molecule to OH-.

OH- is a water molecule that has an extra ion—and thus the term "ionized water" describes the current state of the water. This water, infused with ions, forms a hydroxyl ion—water's natural antioxidant.

Water at the "Fountain of Youth" at Lourdes, France has an alkaline pH of 9.5. This same alkaline range is found at pristine springs and glacial streams around the world.

Hydrogen Water

The term pH is short for "potential of Hydrogen." It's a measure of the amount of hydrogen in any liquid, including, of course, and fundamentally, water. This is important because hydrogen is our fuel—in essence, our Life Force.

Sang Whang in Reverse Aging said water has memory and that this memory is expressed as electrical energy that can be measured in millivolts.

The electrical charge of the hydrogen atoms in water can assume two different forms. One form is hydrogen that has a positive electrical charge, making the water acidic.

The other form is hydrogen that bonds with an oxygen atom. It becomes negatively charged and is alkaline.

In both forms, these atoms or ions (an ion is an atom with an electrical charge), have the capability to bring about chemical reactions. We are chemical organisms, driven by electricity. At the molecular level, trillions of electrically uniting and repelling actions are happening every millisecond of your life.

Therefore, it's not simply a question of whether you choose acidic or alkaline foods and beverages. You're choosing to either add hydrogen and energize your body, or to not augment your fuel, and acidify and deplete your body.

> *"If there is magic on the planet,*
> *It is contained in the water."*
> **Loren Eisley**

Gel Water
The Fourth Phase of Water[1] is the title of Dr. Gerald Pollack's book, and also the basis of his discovery of

and research with exclusive zone, or "EZ" water. The molecular structure of the water is H3O2, and carries a negative charge. This structured, also know as "gel" water is the basis of his astounding, and quite frankly, world changing research.

Fourth phase water is not only the primary molecular composition of the body's cells, it is the means by which living organisms (that includes you and me, my friend) stay hydrated. Yet more wonderful is the fact that you can "make" structured/gel water with chia seeds, which not only hold up to nine times their volume in water, but are also highly alkaline and, *ta-da!* super-bonus, they provide a rich amount of omega-3.

Where do Free Radicals Come From?
Free radicals are produced as a normal part of our bodily processes, for example, food digestion. Normal free radical production is countered by the body producing enzymes to neutralize free radicals.

But the stressors of our current daily lives far, far exceed the ability of our bodies to produce enough enzymes to counteract all of this stress and neutralize the excess of free radicals.

To recap, we have an excess of acidic input from acidic foods, acidic beverages, acidic air, acidic chemicals, as well as acidic, toxic, stress: traffic stress, money stress, family stress, work stress, lack of adequate physical activity stress, over-exerted physical stress, prescribed, acidic drugs, not-prescribed drugs (either over-the-counter or illicit drugs), etcetera.

And there's computer stress which adds double stressors:

1. The stress of EMFs—electro-magnetic frequencies, zinging off a computer screen

2. The stress of the irritation when a computer or a program doesn't work properly, or it's not understood, or you can't communicate with anyone about its non-performance.

There is the no stopping to *"Be In The Moment"* stress.

That's why, in addition to adequate water, which is the most important alkaline substance, you need, too, to supplement your diet with antioxidant foods and antioxidant beverages, and to engage in antioxidant-supporting activities such as yoga and meditation, to neutralize the excess of free radicals so they won't damage your cells.

"In my opinion, the wonder of antioxidant water is its ability to neutralize toxins, but it is not a medicine. The difference is that medicine can only apply to each individual case, whereas antioxidant water can be consumed (by anyone), with amazing neutralizing power."
Prof. Kuwata Keijiroo, M.D.

Uses for Acidic Water
Plants Prefer Acidic Water

Plants have essentially the opposite biology of animals. While a human body needs an alkaline and antioxidant diet, a plant needs an acidic diet. Plants produce oxygen as a byproduct, which animals (that includes humans) use for breath, for energy, for life. Animals produce carbon dioxide as a byproduct, which plants breathe. Thus, plants and animals live symbiotically.

If you water your house plants with an acidic water in the 5.5 pH range, they will thrive. They'll respond with robust oxygen that enhances and detoxifies the air they produce in your home that, in turn, will make you healthier.

Acidic water sprayed on garden plants benefits their health, and repels insects. Garden pests are of the animal kingdom and prefer alkaline water, so acidic water is a natural pest deterrent, without the use of chemicals.

One can only wonder why farmers do not employ acidic water to both grow healthier crops and to deter pests, in preference to contaminating us, the water table, and the entire planet with horrific poisonous chemistry.

The Russians were the first to discover how to make highly acidic water for use on produce. When they developed the highly acidic water, they had a byproduct that they began running tests on, at which point they invited Japanese businessmen to look at their experiments.

It was discovered that the byproduct of the highly acidic water had characteristics of natural spring and glacial stream water. This was when they realized that the "waste product" of highly acidic water for their plants was super alkaline water, full of the natural antioxidant, hydroxyl ions. They then hypothesized that drinking this highly alkaline water would make people healthier.

The Japanese businessmen realized that there was a huge market in Japan for this water treatment, and they developed the technology of the appliance that fits on a kitchen countertop. It has two plates to separate the alkaline and acidic water, and soon the first water ionizer companies were in business supplying the Japanese people with water ionizers. Now, several decades later, home water ionizers are found all around the world.

Other Uses for Acidic Water
In the kitchen, acidic water cleans everything, while preventing food poisoning from bacteria, including e-coli. (Use the same caution with acidic water on granite counters as you do with other cleaners on granite counters.)

Also rinsing your foods in acidic water eliminates bacteria.

Use acidic water as a hand sanitizer and to remove strong odors, such as onion and garlic.

Acidic water cleans scrapes and cuts, and prevents infections. It also alleviates pain and inflammation from minor burns, and aids healing.

Acid water is an astringent, it helps treat acne and other minor skin issues, and makes your skin smooth.

Rinsing your hair with acidic water after shampooing helps prevent dandruff and hair loss.

Bathe your pets in acidic water to give them a healthy, shiny coat!

> *"For many of us, water simply flows from a faucet, and we think little about it beyond this point of contact. We have lost a sense of respect for the wild river, for the complex workings of a wetland, for the intricate web of life that water supports."*
> **Sandra Postel, Last Oasis: Facing Water Scarcity**

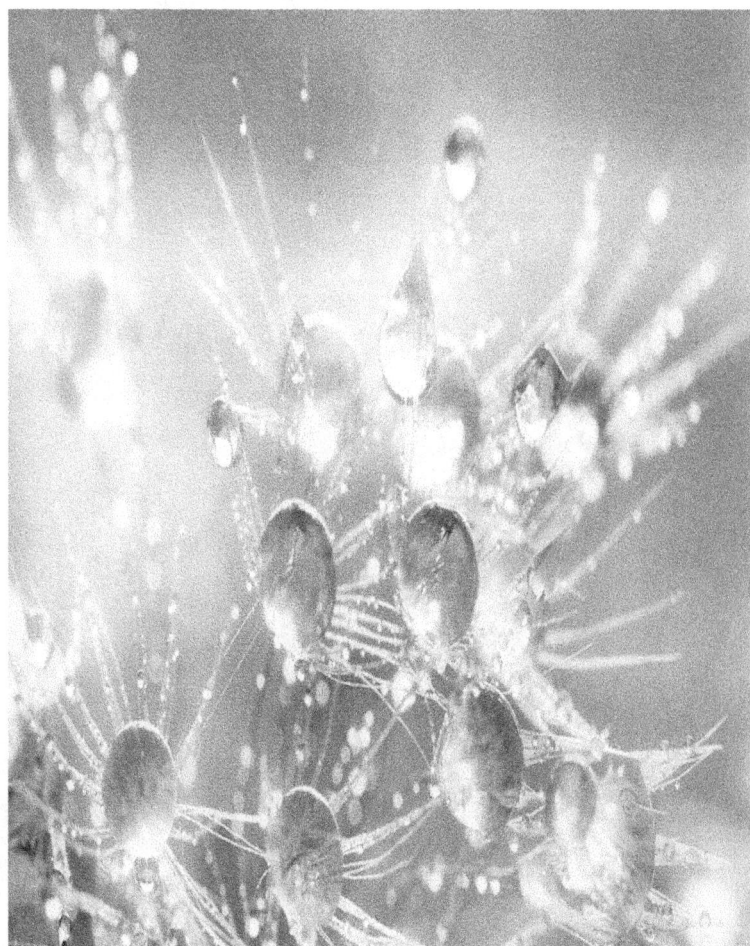

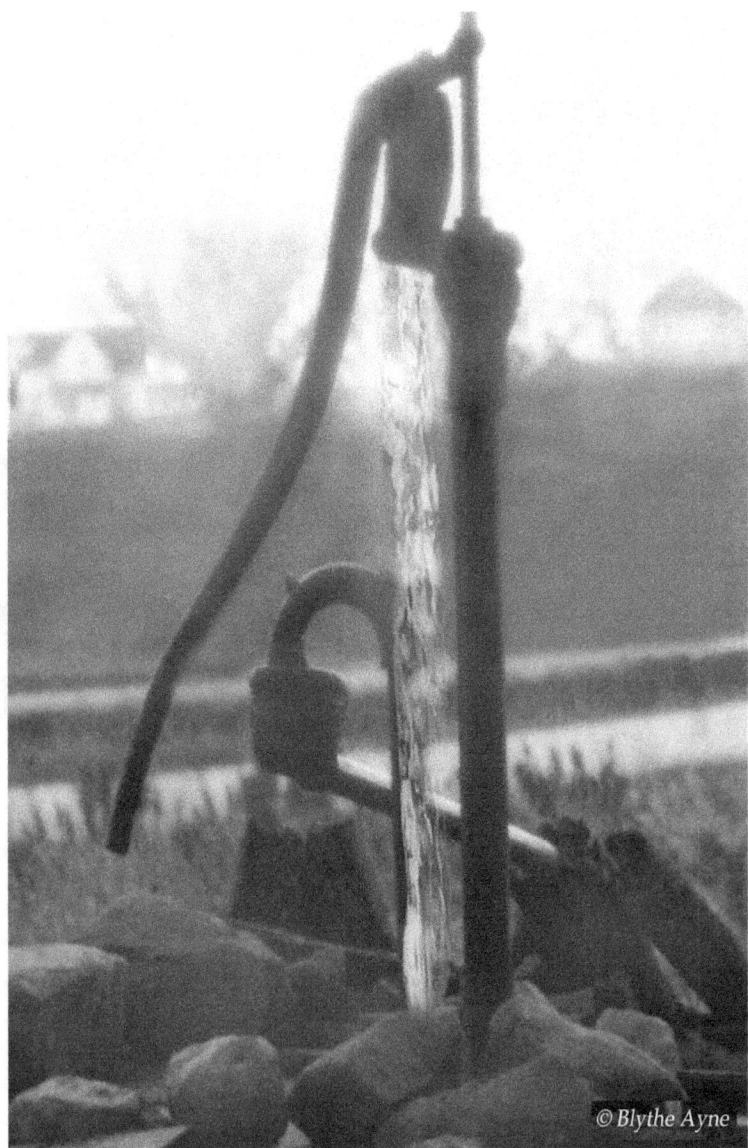

© Blythe Ayne

Chapter 7
Drink More Water

*F*or some people, drinking more water is not easy. The reason so many people give for not drinking more water is the inconvenience of trips to the bathroom. But I trust that this book has made you realize that the benefits of drinking water—a longer and healthier life—far outweigh a small inconvenience.

Start out Your Day with Two Glasses of Water

The Japanese, who have a notable population of the longest-lived and healthiest people on Earth, start the day out, very first thing when they awaken before even brushing their teeth, by drinking down 20 ounces of water. It breaks the night's fasting with an alkaline cleansing that helps clear out the wastes your body has worked hard on all night to remove. It's invigorating and sets the tone of the day.

It's also extremely beneficial to drink a glass of between room-and-body temperature water with a half or a whole lemon squeezed or juiced into it. Drink it down directly once the lemon has been cut, as the phytonutrients are short-lived when exposed to air.

The reason for the tepid temperature of the water is so your body does not have to work to raise the temperature of the water, and you get the full value of the lemon's nutrients, nor are the lemon's delicate nutrients damaged in too-hot water. Drink this lemon water at least 20 minutes away from drinking another beverage or eating. In this way your body can access the full medicinal effect without other digestive processes going on.

As previously mentioned, drink a glass of water before your meals, which curbs over-eating.

Get yourself an attractive, (not PET plastic!) water bottle to carry with you. Or more than one. One for the car, one for the gym, one for the desk, so that you always have water within reach.

And last but not least, simply develop a habit of asking yourself if you've had enough water today.

Water – the Elixir of Life
Water ... no living thing is going far without it! Earth is approximately 70 percent covered in water, and as we are also 70 percent water, Earth's children resemble the parent!

Every little molecule and cell is dependent upon this Wondrous *Elixir of Life*.

In the beautiful work of Dr. Masaru Emoto[1] as shown in his books, *The Hidden Messages in Water, The Miracle of Water, The Secret Life of Water*, he reveals the "heart" of water in its crystalline forms, in photographs.

Dr. Emoto and his researchers discovered the unambiguous response of water to environmental as well as emotional contexts in these crystalline images. His work was explored in the film, *What the Bleep Do We Know?*

Water not only reflects the world it sees in its mirror-like surface, but, on a molecular level, it again reflects the "world" it sees. It's a real-world metaphor for the information we find in books such as *The Holographic Universe* by Michael Talbot[2], exploring the concept that the whole is found in any shard of the parts.

Dr. Emoto's work shows us that when water is in a healthy, negative-ion state, such as mountain streams or spring waters, the crystalline forms of that water are breathtakingly beautiful. When water is taken from stagnant, positive-ion, toxic sources (as in many cities' municipal waters) the crystalline forms of water are distorted and malformed, if, in fact, any crystalline forms manifest at all.

Dr. Emoto and his team also took hundreds of photographs of water that has had intentional thoughts and feelings directed at it. The crystalline forms which materialize in water receiving the thoughts and feelings of "love" and "thank you" are beautifully formed crystals, while the water receiving thoughts and feelings of "hate" formed no crystal at all.

These images can be seen in the book, *The Hidden Messages in Water*, and at: www.masaru-emoto.net/english/water-crystal.html.

"Water has a memory,
and carries within it our thoughts and prayers.
As you yourself are water, no matter where you are,
your prayers will be carried to the rest of the world."
Dr. Masaru Emoto

This quote by Dr. Emoto behooves us to make plentiful our blessings and gratitude, our thoughts, prayers and meditations for ourselves, one another, all creatures, and the planet, in addition to our "message carrier," water.

When you have healthy, ionized, mineralized, de-chemicalized, alkalized water running in your home, not only are you and your family becoming healthier, but that water running down the drain is your small but important contribution to making water healthier on the planet.

Literally, *every little drop helps!*

Your brain is 80 percent water ... give all those firing synapses a healthy, pH balanced, hydrogen-energized, hydrated environment to fire in.

> *The trees reflected in the river —*
> *they are unconscious*
> *of a spiritual world so near to them.*
> *So are we.*
> **Nathaniel Hawthorne**

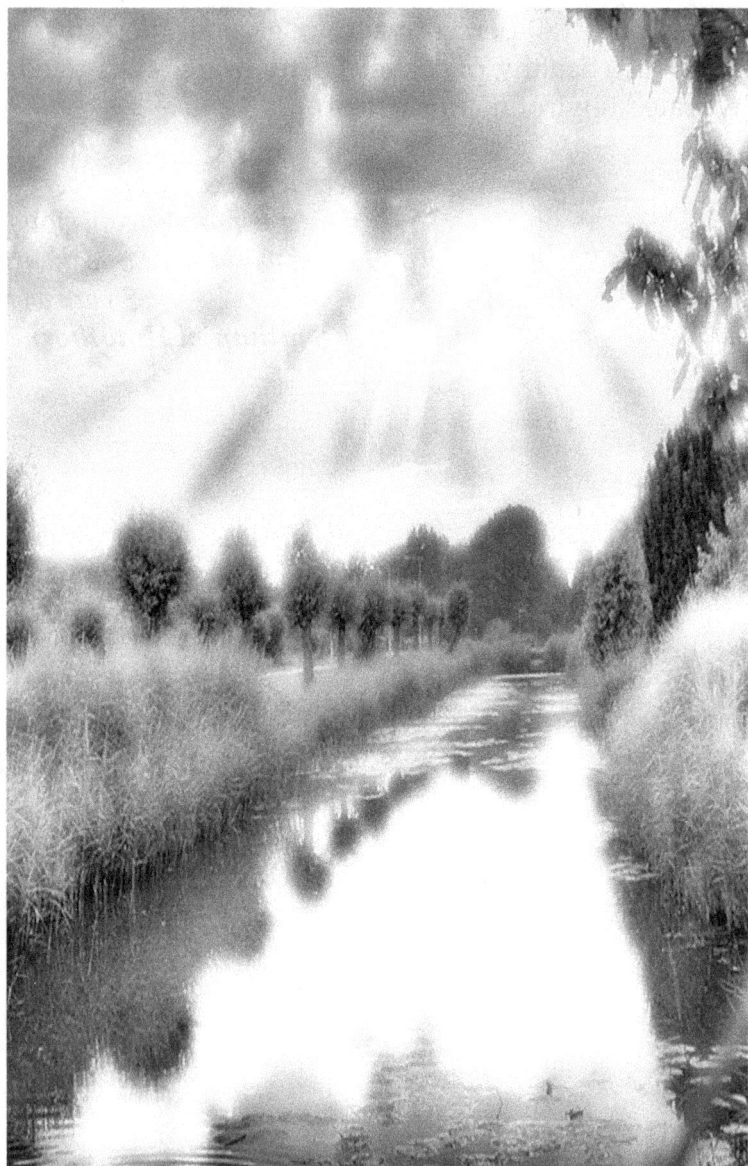

In Closing

"We call upon the waters that rim the earth,
horizon to horizon,
that flow in our rivers and streams,
that fall upon our gardens and fields,
and we ask that they teach us
and show us the way."
Chinook Blessing

*I*f you've read to this point I trust you've had a few insights and intend to establish habits that lead you to assuring that you are well-hydrated and pH balanced.

Is it not particularly compelling that, even as you go mindfully about improving your own health, the benefits are so far-reaching? Not only are you healthier and, consequently, happier, but your pH-balancing life style contributes to the health of the only home we know, our beautiful garden, *EARTH*.

Permit me, after the foregoing science, and the discussion of the various components of the body, and the investigation of sad and heart-breaking diseases from which people are dying many, many years before they ought ... might you indulge me as I move from the prosaic and wax a bit poetic?

I had a thought—maybe it's an insight. Maybe it's even a flash of enlightenment ....

Many, if not most, of the world's cultural histories, religions, belief systems, sacred tribal traditions, mores and folkways, refer to a "place" such as the Garden of Eden. I've contemplated these spiritual locations with curiosity and interest. And while doing so again just now, I had an aha!

The Garden of Eden is the whole Earth.

I know, the recorded details are quite specific, "locating" the Garden of Eden in the midst of four named rivers, and to the "east." But ... what if the four named rivers are meant to represent all of Earth's rivers? What if Earth is to the "east" in the cosmos?

Before you dismiss my thought with a wail of dissent, please appreciate that the only point I'm trying to make is to ponder the fact that you are an overseer of this amazing Garden. Accept that you are called upon to protect, nurture, and love it, just as if it is your own, much-beloved, private, personal garden.

Because it is.

But here's the burning question: Are we doing a good job of it?

There is but one distilled truth in *Save Your Life with the Elixir of WATER*—we are to tend the garden wherein we live, and we are to mindfully tend the individual Garden that each and every one of us is.

Love the Garden of You!
The Garden of You—you are called upon to love the *Garden of You*. In the morning when you wake up, hold the thought of self-love as you drink two glasses of water to break the night's fast in support of your "Morning Body." Throughout the day, mindfully hydrate the beautiful, utterly unique, *Garden of You.*

Your garden will love you in return, with health and tranquility.

* * *

I invite commentary and conversation, dear reader. Agreement, dissent, or questions, all are meaningful. I am inspired by my readers' observations.

You are important to me! May you be well. May you be filled with joy.

Connect with me at:
Blythe@BlytheAyne.com

> *"Till last by Philip's farm I flow*
> *To join the brimming river,*
> *For men may come and men may go,*
> *But I go on for ever."*
> **Alfred Lord Tennyson, The Brook**

Your Gift ....

I'd like to give you a gift for spending this time with me, reading *Save Your Life with the Elixir of Water.*

For your copy of:

Save Your Life with Stupendous Spices

Go to: http://bit.ly/SaveYourLifeSpices

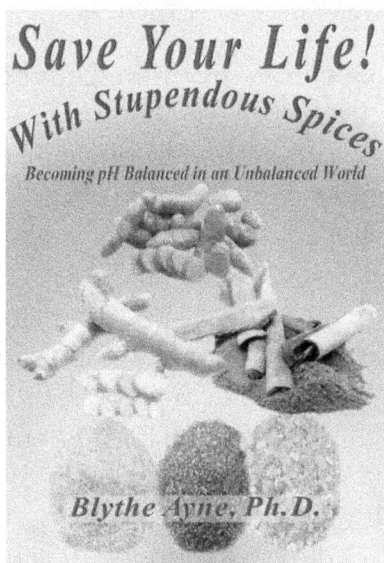

About the Author ....

*H*ere's a thumbnail sketch about me ... I live in a forest with a few domestic and numerous wild creatures, where I create an ever-growing inventory of books, both nonfiction and fiction, short stories, illustrated kid's books, and articles. And I do a bit of wood carving when I need a change of pace.

I received my Doctorate from the University of California at Irvine in the School of Social Sciences, majoring in psychology and ethnography. I've always been filled with wonder contemplating how people think and feel, and what beliefs and actions arise from those thoughts and feelings.

After I submitted my doctoral dissertation, I moved to the Pacific Northwest to write and to have a modest private psychotherapy practice in a small town not much bigger than a village. I had the privilege of working with amazing people, and I witnessed astounding emotional, psychological, and spiritual, healing. It was a wonderful experience.

But after twenty plus years, I realized it was time to put my focus on my writing, where, through the world-shrinking internet, I could "meet" greater numbers of people. *Where I could meet you!*

Your purchase of my work helps support this little corner of the earth, ten acres of natural forest with a year-round stream running through it, and all its resident fauna. All the creatures and I thank you!

I Wish You Happiness, Health, Peace, and Joy,
Blythe

Questions, comments, observations? I'd love to hear from you!:

Blythe@BlytheAyne.com

www.BlytheAyne.com

Resources & References:

Books:

Alkaline Diet for Beginners, Jennifer Koslo, RND, Rockridge Press, 2016

Alkaline Water and the Effects of Drinking it on the Body, Gordon, Amazon, 2015

Alkalize and Ionize, Dr. Theodore A. Baroody, Bis Ediizoni, 2015

Alkalize or Die, Dr. Theodore A. Baroody, Portal, 1991

Cells, Gels and the Engines of Life, Gerald H. Pollack, Ebner and Sons, 2001

Dancing with Water: The New Science of Water, MJ Pangman, Uplifting Press, 2017

H2O, a Biography of Water, Philip Ball, Weidenfeld & Nicolson, 2015

How to Survive in a World Without Antibiotics, Dr. Keith Scott-Mumby, Amazon, 2017

Return to the Joy of Health, Zoltan Rona, and Jeanne Marie Martin, Books Alive, 1995

Reverse Aging, Sang Whang, JSP Publishing, 1991

Running on Water, Walking on Air, Salvatore Parascandolo, Amazon, 2013

Staying Healthy with Nutrition: The Complete Guide to Diet & Nutritional Medicine, Elson M. Haas, Celestial Arts, 2006

The Fourth Phase of Water, Beyond Solid, Liquid, Vapor, Gerald H. Pollack, Ebner and Sons, 2014

The Water Wizard – The Extraordinary Properties of Natural Water, Viktor Schauberger (written circa: 1933), Gill & MacMillan, 1999

Your Body's Many Cries for Water, F. Battmanghelidj, Global Health Solutions, 1995

You're Not Sick, You're Thirsty, F. Battmanghelidj, Grand Central Publishing, 2008

The Hidden Messages in Water, Masaaru Emoto, Atria Books, 2011

The pH Miracle, Dr. Robert O. Young, Grand Central Life & Style, 2010

Water Codes, Carly Nuday, PhD, Water Ink Publishing, 2016

Water Cures, Drugs Kill, F. Battmanghelidj, Global Health Solutions, 2003

Water and the Cell, Gerald H. Pollack and Ivan L. Caameron, Springer, 2007

Websites:
www.statisticbrain.com
www.pollacklab.org
www.waterfyi.com
http://www.ananda.org/Meditation
http://www.thewolfeclinic.com
http://ga.water.usgs.gov/edu/phdiagram.html
http://www.ecy.wa.gov
http://www.alighthere.com/saveyourlifephbalanceattract.html
http://www.freedrinkingwater.com/water-education/quality-water-ph.htm
http://www.mangosteen-natural-remedies.com/benefits-of-drinking-water.html
https://en.m.wikipedia.org/wiki/Human_digestive_system
With thanks to Wiki on many occasions

Podcasts & YouTube Videos:
Green-energy-futures
Alkaway Alkaline Lifestyle
The Real Truth about Health
Dr. Neal Barnard
Dr. T. Colin Campbell
Brenda Davis, RD
Dr. Garth Davis
Dr. Caldwell Esselstyn
Dr. Michael Greger
Dr. John A. McDougall
Dr. Milton Mills
Dr. Gerald Pollack

Notes:

Clinical research by Dr M. T. Morter has shown that if the anabolic urinary and salivary pH measured immediately upon awakening is below 6.8, digestive support must be provided. Clinical studies by Dr. Paul Yanick have confirmed Dr. Morter's findings, recording that intracellular assimilation of nutrients is significantly decreased when the anabolic pH is below 6.8.

Both these researchers have shown that supplementing the diet with alkalizing agents was highly beneficial in elevating the systemic pH by replenishing the alkaline mineral and enzyme reserves. From a preventative perspective, compensation should be made when symptoms are minimal and the anabolic pH is below 7.4 after an Alkaline Load Test.

Diets high in protein, fat, and carbohydrates and low in greens and raw food are stressful to the digestive mechanisms, inhibiting proper digestion and overloading the immune system with incompletely digested macromolecules and toxins, aggravated by the typically high intake of food additives and pesticides common in the Western diet. ("Correlative Urinalysis" by Dr. M. T. Morter).

http://www.earthtym.net/ph-intro.htm
(defunct URL):
"Heavy metals exposure to humans increases the opportunity for parasitic mutation and proliferation, decreases the activity of the immune system, increases

depression leading to slower pro-active behaviors, all of which modifies the pH level considerably in the direction of acidity due to cellular degradation."

KevalaFoundation.org:
"Why are acidic lemons alkaline-producing?
"When we digest lemons they produce alkaline residue. That's why we classify it as an alkaline food. When we digest a food it is chemically oxidized ('burned') to form water, carbon dioxide, and an inorganic compound.

"The alkaline or acidic nature of the inorganic compound formed determines whether the food is alkaline- or acid-producing. If it contains more sodium, potassium or calcium, it's an alkaline food. If it contains more sulphur, phosphate or chloride, it's an acid food."

Ionizers:

A good water ionizer filters out chlorine and leftover pharmaceutical drugs, heavy metals, fluoride and anything else that's nasty in your tap water, while leaving the healthy trace minerals.

The water is filtered and sent to a water electrolysis chamber, which adds ions and antioxidants—this is what happens when water melts from the mountains and flows downstream, bouncing over rocks in the sun. In both cases, the result is clean, antioxidant-rich, ionized water.

There are a number of ionizing products on the market. I encourage you to carefully research these products before purchasing, if you decide to have a home ionizing machine.

GLOSSARY:

Adiponectin - a protein hormone involved in regulating glucose levels and fatty acid breakdown, produced in adipose tissue.

Aerobes - Microorganisms that require an acid, oxygen environment. In the small intestine they prevent the absorption of nutrients.

Amylase - An enzyme, found chiefly in saliva and pancreatic fluid, that converts starch and glycogen into simple sugars.

Anabolic - The synthesis of complex molecules in living organisms from simpler ones together with the storage of energy; constructive metabolism.

Anaerobes - Microorganisms that thrive in an alkaline, oxygen-free environment, they guard against the overgrowth of toxin-producing aerobes.

Benzene - A colorless volatile liquid hydrocarbon present in coal tar and petroleum, used in chemical synthesis. Its use as a solvent has been reduced because of its carcinogenic properties.

Bifidobacteria - Anaerobic bacteria in the gastrointestinal tract.

Bilirubin - An orange-yellow pigment formed in the liver by the breakdown of hemoglobin and excreted in bile.

Carbonic anhydrase - An enzyme that catalyzes the conversion of dissolved bicarbonates into carbon dioxide.

Carcinogens - A substance capable of causing cancer in living tissue.

Catalase - An enzyme that catalyzes the reduction of hydrogen peroxide.

Catabolic - The breakdown of complex molecules in living organisms to form simpler ones, together with the release of energy; destructive metabolism. (Not a bad thing, though it may sound like it. It's simply the opposite process of anabolic. There needs to be a breakdown of materials before there can be a synthesis.)

Chiral - Asymmetric structures—the structure and its mirror image are not superimposable.

Collagen - The main structural protein found in animal connective tissue, from which gelatin is derived.

Cryptosporidium - A parasitic coccidian protozoan found in the intestinal tract of many vertebrates, where it can cause disease.

Endocrine - Of, relating to, or denoting glands that secrete hormones or other products directly into the blood.

Endothelium - The tissue that forms a single layer of cells lining various organs and cavities of the body, such as the blood vessels, heart, and lymphatic vessels.

Epithelium - The thin tissue lining the alimentary canal and other hollow structures.

Exocrine - Relating to or denoting glands that secrete their products through ducts opening onto an epithelium rather than directly into the bloodstream.

Flavones - crystalline compounds occurring in plants. They act as antihistamines, anti-inflammatories, antioxidants, antispasmodic, prevent atherosclerosis, reduce LDL cholesterol, strengthen capillaries, and contribute significantly to cancer prevention. They strengthen the immune system, reduce glucose levels and promote insulin production. How to get them all? Eat every color of fruit and vegetables—the flavones are the green, orange, yellow and red in them.

Flavonoids - plant pigments with a structure based on, or similar to, that of a flavone.

Giardia - infection of the intestine with a flagellate protozoan, which causes diarrhea and other symptoms.

Hyaluronic acid - a mucopolysaccharide that acts as a binding, lubricating, and protective agent.

Interstitial - The small, narrow spaces between tissues or parts of an organ.

Interfacial tissue - Interfaces between various tissues such as skin, fatty and muscles.

Ion - an atom or molecule with a net electric charge due to the loss or gain of one or more electrons.

Lactobacilli - a rod-shaped bacterium that produces lactic acid from the fermentation of carbohydrates.

Legionella - the bacterium that causes legionnaires' disease.

Lumen - the central cavity of a tubular structure in an organism or cell.

Microbiome - The habitat of the microbiota.

Microbiota - The microorganisms in the small intestine.

Mycobacteria - a bacterium of a group causing leprosy and tuberculosis.

Osmosis - a process by which molecules of a solvent tend to pass through a semipermeable membrane from a less concentrated solution into a more concentrated solution.

Phthalates - a crystalline acid derived from benzene, with two carboxylic acid groups attached to the benzene ring.

Phytochemicals (or) Phytonutrients - biologically active compounds in plants, produced by light interacting with earth and water, which has nutritional value.

Polyethylene terephthalate - a synthetic resin made by copolymerizing ethylene glycol and terephthalic acid, widely used to make polyester fibers.

Pseudomonas - a bacterium occurring in soil and detritus, including a number that are disease causing pathogens.

Pyrogens - a substance produced by a bacterium that causes fever when introduced or released into the blood.

Superoxide dismutase - an enzyme that catalyzes the dismutation (simultaneous oxidation and reduction) of the superoxide radical into molecular oxygen or hydrogen peroxide.

Toxins - An antigenic poison or venom of plant or animal origin, produced by or derived from microorganisms and causing disease when present at low concentration in the body.

FOOTNOTES:

Chapter 1:

[1] Peronnet et al. 2012

[2] *Save Your Life with the Phenomenal Lemon & Lime*, Blythe Ayne, Ph.D. – Available in ebook, paperback and hardbound, wherever books are sold.

Chapter 2:

[1] https://en.m.wikipedia.org/wiki/Cerebrospinal_fluid

[2] Newport Natural Health

[3] https://en.m.wikipedia.org/siki/collagen

[4] *The Water Secret: The Cellular Breakthrough to Look and Feel 10 Years Younger,* Dr. Howard Murad

[5] *Save Your Life with the Phenomenal Lemon & Lime*, Blythe Ayne, Ph.D.

[6] https://alkalinenationusa.com/blogs/alkaline-nation-blog/84247617-how-emotions-affect-your-ph-balance

[7] Loughborough University, England

Chapter 3:

[1] *Reverse Aging*, Sang Whang

[2] *Alkalize or Die*, Dr. Theodore Baroody

[3] Hospital Bichat in Paris, France

[4] *https://www.ncbi.nlm.nih.gov/pubmed/ 19083400*

[5] From: *Water for Life*

[6]*https://www.ncbi.nlm.nih.gov/pubmed/16945392*

[7] *https://www.rheumatology.org/I-Am-A/Patient-Caregiver/Diseases-Conditions/Gout*

Chapter 6:
[1] *The Fourth Phase of Water*, Dr. Gerald Pollack

Chapter 7:
[1] *The Hidden Messages in Water, The Miracle of Water, The Secret Life of Water*, Dr. Masaru Emoto

[2] *The Holographic Universe*, Michael Talbot